T0225763

Public Health in China

Volume 4

Series editor

Liming Li, Beijing, China

Public Health in China Series introduces the development and experience in China public health, with comprehensive, objective and accurate data support. It includes 10 volumes, which will be published in 2017 and 2018.

It is a co-publishing series with People's Medical Publishing House (PMPH).

More information about this series at http://www.springer.com/series/15623

Liming Li • Qingwu Jiang

Editors

Introduction to Public Health in China

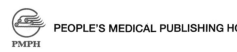
PEOPLE'S MEDICAL PUBLISHING HOUSE
PMPH

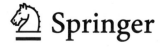
Springer

Editors
Liming Li
Department of Epidemiology
School of Public Health
Peking University
Beijing
China

Qingwu Jiang
School of Public Health
Fudan University
Shanghai
China

ISSN 2520-8365   ISSN 2520-8373   (electronic)
Public Health in China
ISBN 978-981-13-6547-8   ISBN 978-981-13-6545-4   (eBook)
https://doi.org/10.1007/978-981-13-6545-4

© Springer Nature Singapore Pte Ltd. and People's Medical Publishing House, PR of China 2019
This work is subject to copyright. All rights are reserved by the Publisher, whether the whole or part of the material is concerned, specifically the rights of translation, reprinting, reuse of illustrations, recitation, broadcasting, reproduction on microfilms or in any other physical way, and transmission or information storage and retrieval, electronic adaptation, computer software, or by similar or dissimilar methodology now known or hereafter developed.
The use of general descriptive names, registered names, trademarks, service marks, etc. in this publication does not imply, even in the absence of a specific statement, that such names are exempt from the relevant protective laws and regulations and therefore free for general use.
The publisher, the authors, and the editors are safe to assume that the advice and information in this book are believed to be true and accurate at the date of publication. Neither the publisher nor the authors or the editors give a warranty, express or implied, with respect to the material contained herein or for any errors or omissions that may have been made. The publisher remains neutral with regard to jurisdictional claims in published maps and institutional affiliations.

This Springer imprint is published by the registered company Springer Nature Singapore Pte Ltd.
The registered company address is: 152 Beach Road, #21-01/04 Gateway East, Singapore 189721, Singapore

Special thanks go to China Medical Board for funding the publication of this book.

Preface

Public health is the science and practice of preventing and controlling diseases, maintaining and promoting health, enhancing quality of life, and prolonging healthy lifespan. It is also a science and art with population based interventions to achieve its goal through organized efforts of society. Public health in China has developed over 60 years, along with the growth of the People's Republic of China. China's overall health level has reached the average of middle and high income countries. These achievements have been well recognized internationally.

From the founding of New China in 1949 to the economic reform in the late 1970s, China's disease prevention and control system, followed the bio medical model, had been characterized by the planned immunization program and patriotic health campaign, and was supported by preventive medicine education system and epidemic prevention stations across the country. Epidemiology and five major disciplines (food safety, occupational health, environmental health, and school health and radiation safety) comprised the main knowledge system, with the practical work focused on disease prevention and health inspection. This public health system achieved the goal of "wide coverage, high efficiency with low inputs." From that time, China had already established its preliminary health system with "distinctive Chinese characteristics."

The outbreak of severe acute respiratory syndrome (SARS) in 2003 was a turning point in the history of public health in China, which aroused huge concerns from the government, the general public, and the whole society. From then, the government attached great importance to strengthen the disease prevention and control system, which was also leading to the rapid development of public health education, as well as the improvements in public health surveillance and emergency response mechanism. In 2009, a new round of health reform began, highlighting its key objectives of "gradually achieving equitable access to basic public health services." Public health became one crucial component of the health reform tasks with the overall goal of universal health coverage for all.

Over the 60 years, China has made remarkable achievements in the areas such as the national immunization program, maternal and child health, disease surveillance, the establishment of a public health information system and its application, as well as the improvement of people's health, with tremendous experience and best practices being accumulated. In the new era, China starts a new journey towards building Healthy China, which is of great significance for the country's public health development.

In this book, China's public health work is introduced in detail, including its scope and characteristics, its history and evolution, its achievements and experience, as well as the guiding principles for health development, health service system, public health education as well as science and technology of public health. Opportunities and challenges of China's public health are also presented, along with the prospects of future development. We hope the international community will have a better understanding of the history and current situation of China's public health, as well as its achievements and contributions made to date, from reading this book.

I would like to express my sincere gratitude to the members of the Editorial Board for their contributions to, and support for writing, this book. The history of public health in China over the last six decades can be described as a magnificent scroll painting. The narrative of this history, as well as the reflections, was a pioneering and complex task. As such, errors and omissions are inevitable. We welcome comments and criticisms from our readers in this regard.

Beijing, China   Liming Li
Shanghai, China   Qingwu Jiang

Contents

1   Introduction 1
    Liming Li and Qingwu Jiang

2   History and Development of Public Health 13
    Jinling Tang, Fei Yan, and Liming Li

3   Current Situation in China 45
    Liming Li, Guangcai Duan, Haichao Lei, Xiaodong Tan,
    Chun Chang, and Weiyan Jian

4   Public Health Challenges in China 63
    Liming Li, Xiaosong Li, and Bo Wang

5   A Few Thinking About Public Health Development in China 69
    Liming Li, Yu Jiang, and Jun Lv

6   Prospects for Future Development 73
    Liming Li and Hui Liu

Further Reading 81

Contributors

Chun Chang[1] School of Public Health, Peking University, Beijing, China

Guangcai Duan School of Public Health, Zhengzhou University, Zhengzhou, China

Qingwu Jiang School of Public Health, Fudan University, Shanghai, China

Yu Jiang School of Public Health, Peking Union Medical College, Beijing, China

Weiyan Jian School of Public Health, Peking University, Beijing, China

Haichao Lei Beijing Municipal Commission of Health and Family Planning, Beijing, China

Liming Li School of Public Health, Peking University, Beijing, China

Hui Liu Peking Union Medical College, Beijing, China

Xiaosong Li West China School of Public Health, Sichuan University, Chengdu, Sichuan, China

Jun Lv School of Public Health, Peking University, Beijing, China

Jinling Tang The Jockey Club School of Public Health and Primary Care, Chinese University of Hong Kong, Hong Kong, China

Xiaodong Tan School of Public Health, Wuhan University, Wuhan, Hubei, China

Bo Wang Meinian Institute of Health, Beijing, China

Fei Yan School of Public Health, Fudan University, Shanghai, China

---

[1]**Note**: Chinese names are conventionally given with the family name preceding the given names. In this book, we retain that convention for national leaders (for example, President Xi Jinping). Officials, scientists, and others are referred to using the Western convention, in which given names precede the family name (for example, Professor Chun Chang).

Introduction

Liming Li and Qingwu Jiang

1.1 What Is Public Health?

The term "public health" in English refers to the health of the public (or the masses); however, due to the influence from the former Soviet Union, the word "hygiene" (weisheng) instead of "health" has been used in its Chinese translation [1]. The Chinese term weisheng encompasses two concepts in English: hygiene and sanitation. In the modern English dictionary, "hygiene" is defined as "practical actions aimed at keeping the individual person, and his life and work environment, clean for the purpose of disease prevention," while "sanitation" is "systems and equipment in use for maintaining the cleanliness of the environment, particularly for the removal of human excrement" [1]. "Hygiene" is thus focused on the individual's habits, while "sanitation" is about infrastructure and systems aimed at the treatment of garbage and other waste. From the professional perspective in modern society, "hygiene" refers to all practical measures taken by humans in order to protect their health, while "sanitation" refers to measures taken to prevent exposure to harm from waste materials.

In China, the concept of "public health" covers broad and narrow senses [2]: in its narrow sense, it refers to the prevention and control of diseases based on the theories of biology and behavioristics, with epidemiology as its core discipline, which studies three determinants and two influencing factors in the transmission of infectious diseases, the risk factors of chronic noncommunicable diseases, and the strategies to resolve the health issues through high-risk and whole-population

L. Li (✉)
School of Public Health, Peking University, Beijing, China
e-mail: lmlee@vip.163.com

Q. Jiang
School of Public Health, Fudan University, Shanghai, China

© Springer Nature Singapore Pte Ltd. and People's Medical Publishing House,
PR of China 2019
L. Li, Q. Jiang (eds.), *Introduction to Public Health in China*, Public Health in China,
https://doi.org/10.1007/978-981-13-6545-4_1

interventions; in a broad sense, public health is the cornerstone of population health, aimed at promoting the health of entire populations, with sociology and public health as its theoretical basis; and a number of core disciplines are established to collect evidence from multiple perspectives, mainly focusing on health equity, health policy, and environmental impact and through formulating public policies, to ensure the general public's long-term, fundamental health benefits. At the primary stage of socialism, China still needs to address the challenges caused by urban-rural dual structure and the socioeconomic disparities between eastern, central, and western regions. In such a context, China's healthcare reform is intended to provide basic healthcare for all. Public health policy directly affects the people and covers all populations; therefore, to ensure equal access to public health services is a key step toward the goal of China's health reform [3].

The objective of public health is for the health of mankind. Health is a basic human right. It is one key element for sustainable development of a society. Health determinants include human behavior and lifestyles, environmental and biological factors, and the healthcare services. In 1920, Professor C.E.A. Winslow of Yale University defined public health as "the science and art of preventing disease, prolonging life and promoting physical health and efficiency through organized community efforts for the sanitation of the environment, the control of community infections, the education of the individual in principles of personal hygiene, the organization of medical and nursing service for the early diagnosis and preventive treatment of disease, and the development of the social machinery which will ensure to every individual in the community a standard of living adequate for the maintenance of health; organizing these benefits in such fashion as to enable every citizen to realize his birthright of health and longevity [4]." The World Health Organization (WHO) adopted this definition in 1952 [5]. In 1988, Sir Donald Acheson of the United Kingdom gave a short definition of public health as "the science and art of preventing disease, prolonging life and promoting health through the organized efforts of society [6]." In 1995, the US Institute of Medicine (IOM) (now known as the National Academy of Medicine) defined the mission of public health as fulfilling society's interest in assuring conditions in which people can stay healthy [7]. These conditions include working and living environment, lifestyle, and healthcare services. This definition means that public health institutions in the United States have the responsibility to provide healthcare services for millions of people who have been turned away by other healthcare institutions.

In 2003, the Chinese government put forward its own definition of public health at the annual National Health Conference [8]: public health is to prevent disease and promote health through organized efforts of the whole society in improving environment and sanitation conditions, preventing and controlling of infectious and other diseases, developing good personal hygiene and healthy lifestyles, and providing healthcare services. Hence, public health takes social justice as the basis of value, with serving the society as its characteristics, and covering ever-expanding services and objectives, and works toward a common goal of achieving health for all; governments at all levels shoulder the basic responsibilities with the cooperation from all sectors and take the preventive interventions that should be evidence-based.

In summary, the ultimate goal of public health is to promote human health, to prolong life, and to provide healthcare services to cover the whole population. The essential part of public health is to develop public policies and practice health promotion, for which strong government leadership and relevant legislation are needed. Moreover, public health concerns social issues rather than medical and technical issues, with the implication of involving all aspects in the society in the implementation of the measures, requiring social mobilization and multi-sectoral participation. One issue needs to be particularly addressed: public health is an undertaking in need of long-time social return, so a dedicated team of professionals with strong technical and multidisciplinary background is important.

1.2 The Scope of Public Health

1.2.1 A Broad Science: Theories and Disciplines

The study of public health covers broad areas, which expand over time. The key contents include [9]:

- Distribution of disease and health outcome within the population, its influencing factors, and preventive strategies
- Interrelationship of physical and living environment with population health and patterns that reveal the impact of environmental factors on population health and the use of positive environmental factors in the control of negative factors
- The detrimental effects of exogenous factors on human health, biological mechanisms, safety assessment and risk analysis, and the corresponding management measures and laws
- Laws of human nutrition and improvement measures, factors that harm human health and which may be present in foods and the mechanisms of action of such factors, and the subsequent proposal of preventive mechanisms
- Identifying, assessing, predicting, and controlling the impact of poor working conditions on the health of employees
- The relationships between human behavior, lifestyle with health, and patterns in such relationships in search of effective, practical, and cost-efficient interventional strategies, measures, and means of assessment
- Patterns in social factors and individual-group interactions and the corresponding health protection measures
- The physical and mental characteristics and patterns and health needs of mother and infant, of young children and children, of youth, of women, and of the elderly as well as the corresponding health measures to be taken with each group
- Patterns pertaining to social health insurance and insurance activity and the relationship between the two
- Economic activities and economic relations arising from health service delivery, i.e., health-related productive forces and relations of production
- The characteristics and principles of health legislation, relationships, and the establishment as well as implementation of health legislation

- Theories, methods, policies, resources, organization, administration and performance, and the systemic relationships between these elements as pertaining to healthcare management; theories and methods pertaining to the collection, analysis, interpretation, and description of data from healthcare activities
- Processes, patterns, and methods related to information management in healthcare
- Methods and theories for the measurement of the quantity and quality of health-related chemical substances
- Patterns in microbe-environment interactions, the impact on human health, and coping strategies
- Public health is a broad science with its theories in constant development. The key theories include:
- Theories of diseases and influencing factors and theories of etiology and causal inference
- Exogenous chemical toxicity and toxicity; dose and dose-response relationship; mutagenic, teratogenic, and carcinogenic agents; toxicogenomics; systemic toxicology; theories of toxicology management; and risk analysis
- The relationship between man and the environment theories of health risk assessment and the assessment of environmental quality; the function of nutrients and needs, nutrition-related diseases, food safety and the management of such issues, and assessments of food safety
- Theories of occupational physiology, occupational psychology, and occupational pathology
- Theories of health-related behaviors and changes in such behaviors; theories of mutual influence and coordinated development between quality of life, health efforts, population health, and society and the economy
- Health service needs, supply, market, resource procurement and allocation, and costing, as well as related theories of assessment and analysis
- Theories of fund measurement, fundraising payment, and management with regard to social health insurance
- Theories of healthcare system objectives, planning, organization, coordination, control, and performance evaluation
- Theories of the collection, standardized management, statistical description, statistical inference, and utilization of healthcare data
- Theories of quality, quantity, and variation of health-related chemical substances
- Theories of microbial growth, proliferation and death, and the effects of environmental microbes and microbial ecology on human health

The education system of public health and preventive medicine contains nine components as its knowledge base [1]: (1) the epidemiology of disease and influencing factors and causes; (2) the relationship between environmental harmful factors and human health; (3) toxicological knowledge about the toxicity of various exogenous chemicals and their mechanisms of action; (4) knowledge on the nutritional needs of humans and on the health effects of food safety; (5) knowledge about health-related behaviors and influencing factors; (6) knowledge on social factors related to health and health services; (7) knowledge on health, health management, and health policies and regulations; (8) statistical knowledge with regard to the collection, management, description, and inference of health data; and (9) knowledge of the testing and analysis of chemicals and pathogenic microbes.

Public health research adopts the methodologies which include [1]:

(1) Studies at the cellular, molecular, and even more microscopic levels based on molecular biology, molecular genetics, proteomics, cell biology, and chemical physics.
(2) Molecular- and cellular-level research methods for toxicological studies are used together to support the research of organs and biological systems.
(3) Epidemiologists utilizing methods found in biology, psychology, sociology, anthropology, etc., together with methods distinct to the discipline as they study the individual, the group, and the population.
(4) On the global level, methods from geography, ecology, and information science are used.
(5) At all levels, methods from health statistics are utilized in studies.

In China, public health comprises the following disciplines [8, 10]:

(1) Epidemiology and health statistics

Epidemiology is the study of the distribution and determinants of diseases and health within a population. It is also about the development of strategies and methodology to prevent disease and to promote health. Health statistics is a discipline that makes use of theories and methods of probability and mathematical statistics to study the health status of a population as well as to collect, organize, and analyze data from the health service sector, with finally statistical inference with, and the reporting of, such processed data. Epidemiology and health statistics are not only theoretical and applied subjects in public health and preventive medicine but also the essential and core subjects in modern medicine.

(2) Environmental and occupational health

This area is concerned with the study of the impact of the natural environment, the working environment, and living conditions on human health and how to prevent damage to health in these instances. The key tasks for scholars engaging in occupational and environmental health are to identify, evaluate, predict, and control harmful environmental factors; the study of ergonomics and its improvement; the study of the mechanism of action for various harms to health; the search for targets of intervention; and the establishment of preventive strategies for creating better lives and workplace environments. This will help to protect and promote health of the population, contributing to the sustainable development of the country's economy.

(3) Nutrition and food safety

This area comprises two closely linked disciplines: nutrition and food safety. The science of nutrition is to study the biological impact and benefits of nutrients in food as well as other bio-active substances on human health, while food safety is focused on the science of harmful substances that may be found in food and ways of preventing harm to human health by these substances. Nutrition and food safety are an important part of disease control and health monitoring and supervision efforts and play a key role in ensuring the health of the general population, the physical fitness of the population, the enhancement of the body's resistance to disease and harmful elements in the environment, the enhancement of labor productivity, the lowering of disease morbidity and mortality, and the prolonging of longevity.

(4) Population health science

Population health science is concerned with issues that pertain to the development of the population, such as the protection and promotion of both physical and mental health of women, children, and youth. It is concerned with growth and development in the population, the psychological health of the population, the correction of risky behaviors by adolescents, the early prevention of adult diseases, etc. Key areas of research within population health science include the prevention and treatment of common diseases in the area of maternal and child healthcare, infant healthcare, and the health promotion in early life.

(5) Toxicology

Toxicology is the study of all exogenous sources of harm (such as chemical, biological, and physical) to the biological system, as well as the biological mechanisms involved and safety evaluation/risk assessment. The aim and task of toxicology is to study various exogenous chemicals, biological toxins, and physical factors that cause toxicity or harm to the body and to establish the dose-response curves and the mechanism of action for these factors in order to provide the theoretical grounds for the establishment of health standards and preventive measures. Health toxicology is a basic subject in preventive medicine and provides other disciplines with methods. At the same time, health toxicology – an applied science – also has its own theoretical system and research methods.

(6) Social medicine

Social medicine is to study the medical issues from the social perspective and the social issues from the medical perspective and also to propose solutions and strategies from the management perspective. Through the study of interactions between social factors with individual and group health and disease, the study of the health situation in society and its patterns, and the development of social health strategies and health service systems, medical sociology makes a contribution to public welfare by facilitating the delivery of timely, effective, and appropriate health services and improving the health situation in society as well as citizens' health, thereby to maximize health, economic, and social benefits with limited healthcare resources.

1.2.2 China's Public Health Approaches

China's public health strategies cover five stages through individual's whole life course, including newborns and infants (0–1 year old), children (2–14 years old), adolescents (15–24 years old), adults (25–59 years old), and older people (60 years old and above and defined as 65 years old and above in advanced countries). Four public health approaches are taken to address the specific needs of the different groups of population [1, 11].

(1) Preventive health services

Including (1) family planning; (2) maternal and child healthcare; (3) immunization; (4) healthcare for the elderly, such as the prevention of chronic diseases like high blood pressure and cardiovascular and cerebrovascular diseases; and (5) the improvement of healthcare and other health services, such as the advocacy of general medicine services and the prevention of iatrogenic diseases.

(2) Disease prevention (health protection)

Including (1) the control and monitoring of infectious diseases and endemic diseases; (2) the control of harmful elements in the environment (air, water, and noise pollution, as well as food contamination); (3) occupational safety and health; and (4) the prevention of injury and the provision of emergency healthcare.

(3) Health education (health promotion)

Action designed to change the individual's unhealthy behaviors so that the individual will be able to keep healthy by (1) quitting smoking, (2) refraining from excessive alcohol use, (3) eliminating abuse of drugs, (4) maintaining a balanced diet, (5) engaging in physical exercise, (6) living a balanced lifestyle, and (7) reducing mental stress.

(4) Studies of health services

Including (1) the collection and statistical analysis of health-related data; (2) studies on the management of health facilities; and (3) reforms in medical education and professional training.

As the definition of "public health" differs from country to country, the key functions of public health may also be defined differently across different states. In the United States, the core functions of public health are assessment, policy development, and assurance; and in 1995, a list of ten basic public health services was put forward [12]. In the United Kingdom, there are ten major functions for modern public health, and this concept guides the country's public health practice [13]. No matter how "public health" is defined, its functions should cover the following areas [9]:

(1) Health surveillance and analysis

The work of health surveillance involves the establishment and building up of disease information systems (i.e., disease information systems, the collection of data pertaining to the outbreak of the disease) and also includes the monitoring of residents' health needs, lifestyle behaviors, and other factors that may pose harm to their health as well as the identification of health issues and the identification of areas of priority. At the same time, professionals working in this area also make use of data collected for analysis and forecasting for early warning purposes.

(2) Investigation on epidemic outbreaks

This is an essential function of public health that has been in place since the nineteenth century. This area of work comprises the investigation and handling of infectious disease outbreaks as well as the investigation and handling of other unexpected public health incidents such as food poisoning, instances of bioterrorism, nuclear radiation contamination, etc.

(3) Developing and managing disease prevention and health promotion programs

Disease prevention and health promotion programs are key components of public health efforts. These programs include expanded immunization, maternal and child health, tobacco control, etc. In the traditional sense, disease prevention and health promotion programs are generally directly implemented by public health agencies after their establishment. With the development of public service industry, public health agencies can choose to run the program directly or contract out to a third party while still remains the management functions with itself.

(4) Promoting quality and efficiency of public health services

This area of work involves efforts to improve the evaluations of public health programs like disease prevention and health promotion programs, including self-assessments and external assessments; enhancement of the appropriate technical studies; and enhancement of the efficiency of public health services to ensure that all residents would be able to enjoy the right services with cost-effectiveness and at the same time promote the improvement of the quality of health services.

(5) Developing public health legislation and strengthening its enforcement

Apart from the provision or management of the relevant public health programs, another key function in public health is the establishment of the corresponding public health legislation. The establishment of public health legislation or rules and regulations serves to clearly establish the responsibilities of the state and various parties in society, thereby paving the way for further development of public health services. At the same time, work will be done to enhance enforcement and monitoring to ensure the implementation of public health legislation.

(6) Raising public health awareness in the community

The initial objectives of public health were the control of infectious diseases, the improvement of environmental health, and the provision of safe drinking water; built on this basis, the objective expands to reduce health inequity between regions and population groups. All these objectives can be realized only with the increased community awareness on public health, while public health agencies can only serve as organizer and coordinator. Thus, the mobilization of community participation in the identification and resolution of key health issues within the community is now being regarded as a key function of modern public health.

(7) Establishing and maintaining partnerships between governments at all levels, between sectors, and within the health sector

The effectiveness of any implementation of public health, a form of public policy, is dependent on the cooperation and participation of various players in society. The implementation of public health policies hinges upon the understanding of, and support for, the relevant public health topics by the corresponding government agencies at various levels. On the other hand, success also depends on the support provided in the course of policy implementation by the likes of teachers, housing developers, enterprise owners, social workers, etc. In addition, internal cooperation within the health sector should also be strengthened, particularly between those working in clinical health and public health. A more detailed argument for this can be found in *Fixing the Cracks: epidemiology, medicine and the health of the public*.

(8) The development and maintenance of a professional and well-trained team

As public health covers a broad area of issues, the development and maintenance of a professional team that is well-trained and which hails from a diverse array of disciplines is important to the completion of objectives within public health. Disciplines involved include epidemiology, biostatistics, and health management, health promotion, and environmental health.

(9) Innovative studies related to public health policy

As any single disease control or health promotion program is only focused on a particular facet of public health, in general little attention is paid to the development of public health as a whole. Hence, one task in public health is the undertaking of innovative research with regard to the development of public health as a whole as well as on related policies. As society and the economy continue to develop, the substance of public health has also changed over time. In 1998 and 2002, *The Future of Public Health* and *The Future of the Public's Health in the 21ˢᵗ Century* were released respectively in the United States to serve as guidance for the practice of public health [7, 14]. At the same time, research should also be conducted on how to develop health objectives and on how to coordinate all sectors of the society and stakeholders within health sector, within public health sector, to jointly push forward public health work.

1.2.3   Public Health Practices with Chinese Characteristics

When established in 1953, China's disease prevention and control system, which followed the biomedical model, was characterized by the expanded planned immunization program and patriotic health campaign, with support from preventive medicine education and epidemic prevention station. Epidemiology and five major disciplines (food safety, occupational health, environmental health, school health, and radiation safety) comprised the main knowledge system, with the practical work focused on disease prevention and health inspection. This public health system achieved the goal of "wide coverage with low input and high effectiveness [2]." Thus a preliminary health system with "distinctive Chinese characteristics" was established in China.

After 2003 SARS epidemic, the party and the government and the whole society attached great importance to public health. Tremendous efforts were made to strengthen the disease prevention and control system, to boost the public health education, and to build the capacity of health monitoring and emergency response [1]. However, while in the appraisal of the achievements of infectious disease prevention and control, new challenges were imposed on China's health system, for example, the health threats from chronic diseases, environmental health, occupational health, and food and drug safety were largely neglected; the awareness on "broader health concept" in the whole society was still lacking; in addition, when evidence-based health services and decision-making became increasingly important, its application in public health and public health policy-making became an urgent task for China in the future [15].

China's public health has developed for over six decades; its experience could be summarized as: "political commitment, policy support, population-based strategy, prevention first, social mobilization, community participation, appropriate technology, science and technology support, community-based intervention and sufficient funding." These can be further explained as below:

- Public health is a public welfare undertaking. It is indispensable of government leadership and support, as well as a favorable policy and legislation environment.
- The principle of "prevention first" has been implemented in the 60 years. It is proved that pollution-based intervention is the most effective way to prevent disease and reduce the incidence of diseases.
- Public health is for the health of all, involving various sectors such as health, agriculture, environmental protection, education, and technology. It needs social mobilization and multi-sectoral coordination; it also needs to raise public health awareness and promote healthy behaviors through community participation.
- With the rapid development of science and technology, public health professionals are also exploring new knowledge and skills and developing new technologies appropriate for population use, so that effective interventions could be truly implemented to serve the population.
- The concerns from government and all societies, with their financial inputs, are the basic guarantee for the sustainable development of public health.

References

1. Li L, Jiang Q. Theory and practice of public health in China. Beijing: People's Medical Publishing House; 2015.
2. Li L. Reconsideration on 60 years of public health in China. Chin J Public Health Manag. 2014;30(3):311–5.
3. Chinese Academy of Medical Sciences. China medical reform development report (2016). Beijing: Peking Union Medical College Press; 2016.
4. Gatseva PD, Argirova M. Public health: the science of promoting health. J Public Health. 2011;19(3):205–6.
5. World Health Organization. New challenges for public health: report of an interregional meeting. http://apps.who.int/iris/bitstream/handle/10665/63061/WHO_HRH_96.4.pdf
6. Durham University, World Health Organization. Strengthening public health capacity and services in Europe. http://www.euro.who.int/__data/assets/pdf_file/0007/152683/e95877.pdf
7. Institute of Medicine. The future of public health. Washington: National Academies Press, 1988.
8. Li L. An introduction to public health and preventive medicine. Beijing: People's Medical Publishing House; 2017.
9. Lu J, Li L. The basic functions and scope of modern public health system. Chin J Public Health. 2007;23(8):1022–4.
10. Chinese Preventive Medicine Association. Report of academic developments in public health and preventive medicine (2014–2015). Beijing: Chinese Science and Technology Press; 2016.
11. Li L. Challenges facing public health in China in the 21st century, and countermeasures. Chin J Health Educ. 2003;19(1):5–7.

12. The Core Public Health Functions Steering Committee. The essential services of public health.   http://publichealthne.org/phan-sections/public-health-education-section/marketing/ essential-services-of-public-health/
13. Sir Donald Acheson, Department of Health and Social Security, Great Britain. Public Health in England: the Report of the Committee of Inquiry into the Future Development of the Public Health Function. London: H.M.S.O; 1988.
14. Institute of Medicine. The future of the public's health in the 21st century. Washington: National Academies Press; 2002.
15. Li L. 60 years of public health in China: achievements and prospects. Chin J Public Health Manag. 2014;1:3–4.

History and Development of Public Health

2

Jinling Tang, Fei Yan, and Liming Li

2.1 Public Health from Ancient to Modern Times

2.1.1 Origins of Public Health

Public health is based on preventive medicine; the latter is an integral part of medical science. Medical science is concerned with diseases, the diagnosis, treatment, and rehabilitation of patients. Where there were written accounts on human history, there were records on diseases. Man's understanding on diseases was also a part of the history of human civilization. Before the advent of modern society, diseases were usually regarded as the results of God's will, destiny, and morals, and people always mixed diseases with evil hearts and treatment of diseases with witchcrafts and religion—one evidence is that till now we still call medical science a "temple of God."

The Greek physician Hippocrates (460–377 BC), "the father of modern medicine," put forward "the theory of bodily humors" to explain diseases. In his opinion, the human body was made up of four "humors": blood, phlegm, yellow bile, and black bile, with varying combinations of which causing various health conditions. He saw disease as a phenomenon in progress and believed that physicians ought to treat patients rather than diseases. Hippocrates changed the belief that diseases were caused by superstition and gods; he proposed that while treating

J. Tang
The Jockey Club School of Public Health and Primary Care, Chinese University of Hong Kong, Hong Kong, China

F. Yan
School of Public Health, Fudan University, Shanghai, China

L. Li (✉)
School of Public Health, Peking University, Beijing, China
e-mail: lmlee@vip.163.com

© Springer Nature Singapore Pte Ltd. and People's Medical Publishing House, PR of China 2019
L. Li, Q. Jiang (eds.), *Introduction to Public Health in China*, Public Health in China, https://doi.org/10.1007/978-981-13-6545-4_2

patients, the effects of patients' individual characteristics, environmental factors, as well as lifestyles should be considered.

The discovery of pathogenic microorganisms has promoted further awareness of disease and brought medicine into the field of science [1]. Italian physician Girolamo Fracastoro (1483–1553) proposed the concept of the "spores of disease," wherein disease is caused by external factors ("spores") and may be transmitted either directly or indirectly. Austro-Hungarian M.A. Plenciz (1705–1786) proposed that disease was caused by a live object and that every type of infectious disease was caused by a distinct type of such objects. In the year 1676, the Dutchman Antony van Leeuwenhoek (1632–1723 CE) invented the microscope, which was capable of magnifying objects 266 times. With this microscope, he discovered a number of tiny living things that are invisible to the naked eye, thus proving the scientific evidence of the existence of these living objects.

During the reign of the Emperor Qianlong of the Qing Dynasty in China (1736–1795), the poet Shi Daonan described in *Tian YuJi* numerous plague outbreaks and also pointed out that the rats caused these outbreaks. He wrote: "Dead rats in the east, / Dead rats in the west! / The sight of dead rats makes one shudder, /Days after the passing of the rats, large numbers of men falter. /Under a gray sky and cloudy days, /Countless people die away. / Three men walk together, and in less than ten steps two have fallen forever! /No cries are heard when one dies in the night, for the demon of pestilence has weakened the light. /All of a sudden it all goes dark, leaving man, ghost and coffin in need of spark. / The crows caw incessantly, and the air is filled with the sounds of dogs howling. / Men look like apparitions, while the demon has robbed men's spirits. / Most men one meets in the day are ghosts, yet one wonders if one has met a human when running into another at dusk. / The ground is covered with corpses, and there is no sign of life; human bones become wind-worn over time. / There in the fields are crops to be reaped by none; and officials have no one to go to for tax. / I hope to ride the Heavenly Dragon to see the God and Goddess in Heaven, and beg them to spread their heavenly serum and milk upon the earth, so that spring will return and the dead may come to life again." This is the description of the sad sights witnessed during the plague outbreaks of 1792–1793 CE.

In the publication of Ming Dynasty, the *Compendium of Materia Medica*, Li Shizhen (1518–1593) wrote that patients who had their clothing held over steam did not contract illnesses. This is clearly a record of the process of sterilization. Numerous records show that during the reign of the Emperor Longqing of the Ming Dynasty (1567–1572 CE), inoculation was already widely used against smallpox. The procedure was later adopted by Russia, Korea, Japan, Turkey, England, etc.

From above, we can see public health originated from evolution of human society and the scientific advancement [2]; it is a science and art of human being's longtime battle against diseases. In its Constitution, the WHO states that "health is a state of complete physical, mental and social well-being, and not merely the absence of disease or infirmity [3]." Nowadays, what people need on public health has shifted from "diseases prevention and control" to "promotion of health."

2.1.2   Public Health into Civilized Society

Entering into the civilized society, in order to prevent and control infectious diseases, people started to conduct quantitative observations on the health of the individual and the population [4]. For example, in the seventeenth century, John Graunt studied the distribution and patterns of death; in the eighteenth century, Pierre Charles Alexandre Louis and William Farr proposed a series of important concepts for epidemiology as well as introduced the use of statistics into the field of public health; in 1796, Edward Jenner came up with the inoculation method for smallpox, paving the way for the scientific study of active immunization to prevent infectious diseases. Between 1848 and 1854, John Snow surveyed and analyzed the cholera epidemic in London, coming up with methods of field survey, analysis, and control for the field of epidemiology.

At the same time, advancements in the fields of physics, chemistry, biology, etc., as well as in measurement techniques, also promoted studies of the relationship between the natural and living environments with population health into a period of rapid development. Bernardino Ramazzini first reported diseases like silicosis and lead poisoning, while Percival Pott wrote of the cause-effect relationship between exposure to polycyclic aromatic hydrocarbons and cancer. Claude Bernard studied the mechanism of action for carbon monoxide poisoning and laid down the foundations of occupational toxicology together with François Magendie and Mateu Orfila. Human understanding of the chemical makeup of food and the human body contributed to basic concepts and fundamental theories in nutritional science, while knowledge of harmful factors in the workplace led to basic theories of occupational health and occupational medicine. In the nineteenth century, Louis Pasteur established the germ theory of disease.

By the late nineteenth century to the early twentieth century, mankind had achieved remarkable progress by successfully combating the deadly infectious diseases such as smallpox, cholera, plague, and diphtheria and advancing in the areas of environmental health, occupational health, nutrition and food safety, maternal and child health, and adolescent health. Built on these, a system of public health theories and population-based preventive interventions has been established, with the government taking accountability of providing essential clinical and public health services for all population and also providing appropriate technology for public health work.

2.1.3   Public Health into Modern Age

By the middle of twentieth century, public health has developed into a series of disciplines: for example, epidemiology, which studies public health methodologies, from the spreading to the distribution of diseases, covering not only infectious diseases but all diseases and health challenges; toxicology, which raised safety standards, exposure biomarkers, effect biomarkers, and susceptibility biomarkers, being widely used in the identification and study of environmental factors and health; environmental medicine, which allowed researchers to study the chronic effects on health of harmful factors in the environment, such as mutations, carcinogenic effects, and teratogenic effects; the research of behavioral science in medicine which has laid the theoretical foundation for health education and health promotion created a new field to study the relationship between human behavior and lifestyles with health and diseases; the development of social science, integrated with public health, led to a new discipline of social medicine with the objective of uncovering the relationship between population health with various macro and micro social factors; the advancements in economics, public policy, and the science of management, integrated with public health, promoted the theories and practices of health economics, health policy, and health management.

As early as 1932–1938, Dr. Chen Zhiqian implemented a community-based pilot in Ding County of Hebei Province to explore the primary healthcare system. His efforts were a great boost for China's health development. In 1940s, WHO's revolutionary definition of health promoted the shift of medical model for disease prevention—from biological measures to social and behavioral interventions, from purely passive prevention to active population-based prevention. The term "preventive medicine" began to be used in North America, where the concept of the "three-level prevention of disease" also came into being. Based on their knowledge of the importance of social factors to health, public health scholars focused on the significance of the social environment and policies to health and proposed the ecological model to public health. Until 1986, the Ottawa Charter for Health Promotion highlighted the governments' leadership role in health, including the importance of community development and public participation. This marked the beginning of the "Modern Public Health Age," in which preventive services provided during the life course, as well as before and after diseases, became the core study contents of achieving universal health for all.

Advances in public health methodologies and technologies have facilitated the modern public health development. For example, the ability of sanitary chemical analysis techniques to detect and track constant, trace and ultra-trace amounts, from composition to morphology, from the macro to the micro, from the whole to the discrete level, both statically and dynamically has allowed researchers to engage in the high-throughput screening of harmful chemical factors and the analysis of quantitative structure-activity relationships. In the area of health microbiology, the research focus is not only on pathogenic microorganisms but also on the growth, reproduction, variation, patterns of replacement, and interactions of microbes and microbial populations under microecological conditions, as well as the interactions between microbes and microbial population and the human body. In particular, technological advances in molecular biology have greatly promoted the development of public health in all aspects with in-depth research at the genetic and protein-molecule level. Advances made in the areas of statistics, computing, and information technologies and the application of these disciplines to public health have led to the broad use of multivariate models, multilevel models, structural-equation models, and other mathematical models in public health research.

Technologies like the geographic information system (GIS) have allowed public health researchers to carry out even more precise quantitative studies of population health issues at the macro level, while developments in the areas of monitoring technologies and the emergence of large-scale databases have enabled the study of human health and environmental systems from the molecular level to the ecology as a whole by public health and preventive medicine researchers.

Public health is a booming science within the broad human health studies, with its theories and practices making tremendous progress so far. With the rapid socioeconomic development and drastic changes worldwide, mankind is facing new and emerging public health challenges: lifestyle changes, global warming, changes in pathogenic microbes, the use of chemical products in large quantities, the industrial production of food, worsening environmental pollution, population flows, the exchange and connection of peoples, the swift spread of infectious diseases worldwide, population aging and frequent public health emergencies, and so on [5]. In order to tackle these issues, public health has shown a trend with broader perspective, more disciplines and technology integration, deeper exploration at micro level, and bigger information integration, while the disciplines of public health and preventive medicine will also be expanded to new areas as well.

2.2   Public Health from Ancient China to New China

2.2.1   Philosophy in Ancient China

Chinese history of public health can be traced back to thousands of years ago. The traditional concept of "Five Elements" in Taoism is a systematic theory that has been widely used in traditional Chinese medicine. The *Huangdi Neijing*, or *Inner Canon of the Yellow Emperor* or *Esoteric Scripture of the Yellow Emperor*, compiled around 500 BC, describes the Five Elements theory, including the evolution process of the *yin* and *yang* elements. In theories of traditional Chinese medicine, it was held that natural phenomena could be accounted for by changes in the "Five Elements," which are wood, fire, earth, metal, and water. These phenomena also had the power to affect man's fate and at the same time make up the endless cycle that is the cosmos.

In the *Huangdi Neijing*, it was stated that "The sage does not cure the sick, but prevents illness from arising, not govern chaos, but prevents chaos from arising." "To treat disease and chaos after they have already occurred is like digging a well when one is thirsty, and akin to forging an awl when the occasion for a fight arises. It is far too late!" The control of future disease as referred to here is disease prevention. It was advocated that man can maintain healthy beginning with his lifestyle, through a good diet and exercise and through the management of his mental health so that "he would be full of righteous *qi* and cannot be violated by external evil." We can say that the *Huangdi Neijing* laid the foundation for early philosophical thought on public health.

The impact of "Five Elements" on health, taking the water as an example, can be traced back to the ancient records in *Zuozhuan* as early as 585 BC. "The land at Xunxia is not like that of Xintian, where the soil is good and the water is deep. It may be occupied without fear of disease. There are the Fen and the Kuai rivers to carry away the evil airs; and the people, moreover, are docile. It offers advantages for ten generations. "The "evil airs" here refers to filth. Clearly, it was already known then that dirty water that has accumulated can lead to disease and that discharge of filthy water can insure human health. The *Yangsheng Leizuan* written in the Southern Song period (1127-1279) made the connection even clearer: "Keeping ditches dredged and homes clean and free of evil airs can keep the plague at bay. "These records make it clear that the ancients' thought of sewage treatment was from the perspective of safety, disease prevention, and the prevention of accidents. There had also been a number of attempts and innovations in ancient China in terms of health-related engineering and technologies. Archaeological research shows that city planning and health facility standards in the Tang Dynasty capital of Chang'an were world-leading in their time: there were public lavatories in Chang'an as well as dedicated lavatory-maintenance personnel. The streets were broad spacious, with ditches established on both sides. A ditch excavated along Zhuque Street in what is Xi'an today measured 3.3 m wide and 2.3 m deep. Brick-lined drainage channels ran under the streets in both the eastern and western sides of the city and were connected to the ditches dug by the sides of the streets.

China knew the importance of quarantine in early time. Since the Qin Dynasty (221–206 BC), the "Sick House" system was established. The *Biography of Narendra-yaśas* records that in 557, Indian monk Narendra-yaśas built a "sick house" for lepers at Xiangquan Temple in Henan. It was stated that the sick house "accepted those afflicted with pestilence and disease, with men and women housed in separate quarters; and clothing, food, bedding and medical care were provided to these sick people by the temple staff." Since then, the practice of "sick houses" operated by temples and monasteries continued for three centuries until 845, when the Tang Emperor Wuzong ordered that the function be taken over by local governments.

2.2.2 Early Practice in Ding County

In 1915, epidemiologists Wu Liande and Yan Fuqing organized a public health committee and asked to integrate health education into the mission of the Chinese Medical Association. A plague in the northeast in 1917 killed over 60,000 people and led to the establishment of the Central Bureau for the Prevention of Infectious Diseases in 1919. However, the public's awareness on diseases was still very low. Public health was largely neglected in China's warlord's era before 1949.

It is nevertheless worth noting the experience of Ding County in Hebei Province as an instance of early practice of public health in China. In the 1920s, the Peking Union Medical College (PUMC) embarked on the task of public health education and opened its first health affairs office in Beijing which covered a population of

50,000 persons. In 1928, cooperated with the Association for the Promotion of Mass Education founded by Yan Yangchu, Chen Zhiqian, Chinese public health pioneer, chose Ding County to pilot community healthcare system. He conducted China's first rural healthcare experiment during 1932–1938, which became the first attempt in the research of medical education in China's medical history. The pilot also promoted the local health development. With the support from John B. Grant, Chen Zhiqian established the health agencies at three levels in Ding County: the county, district, and village levels, thus establishing for the first time a "healthcare network" [6]. The implementation of this system, which could be applied to different socioeconomic areas, was widely recognized in China and abroad. However, the pilot had to stop after the outbreak of the Sino-Japanese War in 1937.

In China's public health and primary healthcare history, this so-called Ding County model was referred to Chen Gungqian's great innovation between 1932 and 1938 [7]; he established the "three-tiered rural healthcare network" after detailed surveys of the county and applied modern western medicine and academic knowledge of public health and health education to the specific circumstances of China's villages. At that time, Chen believed that "the strength of any nation is rooted in its general public, thus the people, not just a few in power, should enjoy the best healthcare services [8]." He believed that it was not enough to rely on the existing model wherein missionaries and physicians would open hospitals in the cities and wait for patients to come to them. Both treatment and prevention were needed in Ding County, and medical knowledge would never reach the rural areas through hospitals alone. A greater focus on disease prevention was needed. Chen proposed four principles to be considered when seeking to resolve the issue: (1) healthcare services should be grounded on specific local needs and should be feasible with local conditions; (2) the healthcare system should be locally financed, which required the training of local health workers and reduction of the economic burden of rural residents; (3) a bridge should be established between urban and rural areas so that the modern medicine widely used in the cities can be applied for the rural population; and (4) the community was accountable for the operation and sustainability of the system. Based on these four principles, he designed a comprehensive rural healthcare system (Fig. 2.1).

First, each village identified a village health officer responsible for providing healthcare services for his/her village. The village health officer should be selected among the graduates of the local village school and should also meet the following criteria: passionate, honest and reliable, healthy, and aged between 20 and 35. Before being officially appointed, the health officers must undergo 10 days of basic medical training at a health center. His responsibilities included promoting awareness of disease prevention in his free time, performing inoculations, disinfecting well water, treating trachoma and tinea capitis using available medical supplies, performing first aid for the injured, making improvements to the home well and lavatory as demonstration for the community, and performing birth and death registrations for the village. Physicians should provide guidance to village health officers, particularly in the use of medication to prevent treatment errors. During lull periods in spring and winter, the physicians would hold tea parties to

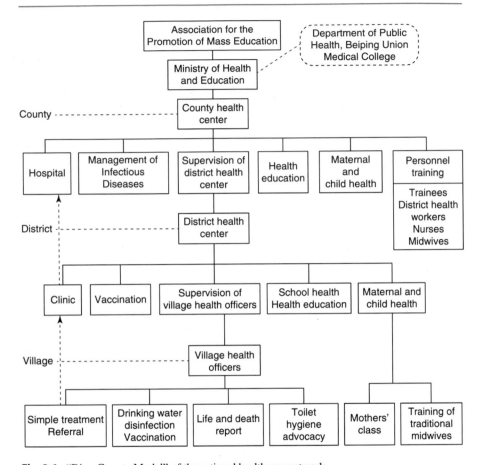

Fig. 2.1 "Ding County Model" of three-tiered healthcare network

keep in touch with each other. Health-related reading material would also be given out at these tea parties to aid in knowledge acquisition. In this way, village health officers could take care of common diseases in the village and then refer patients with diseases that they were unable to handle for treatment at the district or county health center.

Second, to establish district health centers which covered residents of a population of 30,000 of 20 villages, each district health center should have one physician, one nurse, and one assistant. The key responsibilities of the district health center were as follows: train and supervise village health officers, with its physician making field visits to the village at least once every 6 months and health officers making work reports and exchanging their experiences at health center meetings at the same interval; hold daily outpatient clinics for patients, especially patients referred to the center by health officers; responsible for school health and health education; and responsible for the prevention of acute infectious disease. The district health center received patients referred by village health officers and patients with more severe ailments to the county health center. The district health center provided strong support to village health officers and helped them to gain the trust of the villagers.

Third, a county health center, covering 100 villages, was to be established. The county health center was responsible for the management of the health efforts for the entire county and had a leading role in the entire three-level healthcare network. The center had five key responsibilities: (1) the treatment of patients with more severe ailments—in a 30-bed facility with equipment more advanced that what was being used at the district level—for a population of 400,000; (2) dedicated center administrative personnel were to coordinate health agencies and to contact administrative personnel and other relevant local contacts across the county during the outbreak of major infectious diseases such as smallpox and cholera, as well as to manage epidemic response; (3) the center was responsible for the disbursement of a research grant to the health center as well as the procurement of educational materials; (4) the central management of medications across the county to prevent waste and fake drugs; and (5) provide medical school graduates with internship opportunities and at the same time train nurses and assistants. The staff of the county health center include one male physician, one female physician, two assistant physicians, eight nurses, one pharmacist, one inspector, a secretary, and six assistants. There were 50 beds in the center for hospitalized patients. In 1933 alone, a total of 778 patients were hospitalized at the center, with 67.8% male and the rest, female.

The Ding County pilot was a useful experiment to tackle health challenges in resource constrained rural areas of China. A great number of rural residents were able to access to basic healthcare and health protection with the available conditions. This heralded a new era in the history of healthcare in China. The operation cost of the system was low: apart from cost incurred from the annual training of village health officers, each year, medical expenses came up to a total of 35,000 Yuan and less than 1 Jiao annually per person. Statistics from 1931 showed that medical expenses stood at 120,000 Yuan and 3 Jiao annually per person. The average medical care expense per person per year had been reduced by two thirds, bringing great benefit to rural residents. The district health center charged a fee of only five copper coins per visit, while the daily ward rate at the county health center was only 40 cents. These were prices that rural residents could afford, and hence they were able to receive timely and proper treatment for their ailments. By 1935, the Ding County System expanded to cover six districts or half of all villages within the county. In 1935, 220 village health officers performed first-aid services and treated patients on 137,183 occasions and vaccinated 140,000 persons. District health centers treated patients on 65,000 instances, while the county health center saw a total of 626 persons warded and 259 surgical operations performed. Knowledge of health issues among rural residents was significantly enhanced, and they were no longer threatened by illnesses such as neonatal tetanus, puerperal fever, smallpox, and black fever. Instances of various infectious gastrointestinal ailments also declined in number. The Ding County System was even tested by the 1934 Northern China cholera outbreak. Only a few cases were reported across the county, and no fatality was recorded. Smallpox, a disease that had plagued the people for thousands of years, was declared as "eradicated" in Ding County in 1936.

The Ding County has successfully explored a rural public health mechanism and created a model of effective three-tiered system with concerted efforts and coordination of village health officers, district health centers, and country health centers. It was a model characterized by "low level and high efficiency." The system showed how highly impoverished Northern China villages could be provided with modern healthcare services and how to avoid the pitfalls or inadequacies that had already been seen in Soviet Union, the former Yugoslavia, India, etc. Because of this, the Ding County System drew the attention from China and abroad. The League of Nations conducted a field visit to Ding County and invited Chen Zhiqian to talk about his experience in the USA. Within China, the Ding County System was soon adopted in Jiangning and Wuxi on an experimental basis. The Republican Government in Nanjing also decided to duplicate Ding County System model nationwide in 1934. In the late 1940s, the Joint Sino-China Committee for the Rejuvenation of Rural China, which was co-founded by Yan Yangchu, implemented a program in Sichuan Province aimed at enhancing rural health agencies and a tap-water program and anti-malaria and anti-schistosomiasis programs in Taiwan. The committee trained public health personnel at the county and township levels in both provinces, which followed the pilot of Ding County System. The three-tiered healthcare system established in Ding County marked a milestone in the history of public health in China and provided important practical experience for public health researchers and practitioners in the world. Built on it, China continued the development of its rural three-tiered health service network (Fig. 2.2) in the 1950s and then in the late 1960s, the establishment of the wider rural cooperative medical system.

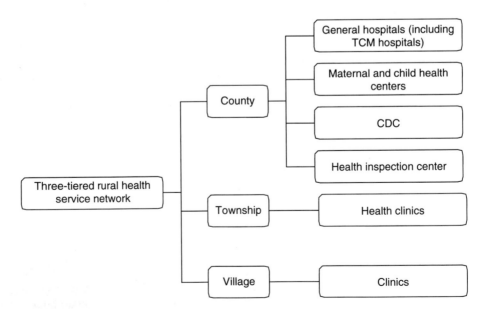

Fig. 2.2 China's three-tiered rural health service network

2.2.3   After the Founding of New China in 1949

(1) Institution Setup (1949–1956)

In line with the Soviet Union's model, in January 1953, the State Council approved the establishment of Epidemic Prevention Station at the provincial, prefectural (city), and county levels across China. In the same year, the National Patriotic Health Campaign Committee Office was established. In 1954, the Ministry of Health released the guidelines for Epidemic Prevention Stations, defining prevention, routine monitoring, and management of infectious diseases as the key responsibilities. By the end of 1956, Epidemic Prevention Stations were set up at the prefectural (city) and county levels in most of the 29 provinces, along with the railway system and large factory and mining enterprises.

At the same time, a series of technical agencies for specific disease prevention and control were established between 1953 and 1963, which covered parasitic diseases, endemic diseases, schistosomiasis, sexually transmitted diseases, leprosy, malaria, tuberculosis, and other infectious diseases. These agencies, together with Epidemic Prevention Station, preliminarily formed China's disease prevention and control system with a focus on five major diseases, which laid a solid foundation for China's infectious disease prevention and control.

(2) Initial Development (1957–1976)

In 1964, the Ministry of Health issued the *Regulations on Epidemic Prevention Station (Trial)* and clearly defined its nature as a public institute with the four key tasks of "Organization, guidance, monitoring and supervision, and law enforcement." In December, the Central Institutional Organization Commission and the Ministry of Health jointly released the *Regulations on the Organization and Staffing of the Epidemic Prevention Station*. These policies standardized the development of Epidemic Prevention Station. Until the end of 1965, 2499 stations were set up across the country, which was 15 times more than that in 1952.

China's Cultural Revolution, which began in 1966, had certain effects on the work of Epidemic Prevention Station. However, during this period, China had gradually established a three-level medical and preventive healthcare network and a cooperative medical system in its rural area. The network, composed of county health facilities, township hospitals, and village clinics, provided an effective platform for disease prevention and control work in rural China and made contribution to its further development.

(3) Restructuring (1977–1997)

In 1979, the Ministry of Health issued its *National Regulations for Epidemic Prevention Station*, outlining the principles for its tasks, organizational structure, responsibilities, and workforce and operating approaches. In 1982, while comprehensively summarizing the experience of the nation's epidemic prevention stations, the Ministry of Health decided to establish China Center for Preventive Medicine (later renamed the Chinese Academy of Preventive Medicine). This marked the formation of a national system of disease prevention and control that operated at various levels, from the center at the national level to epidemic stations at provincial, prefectural, county levels, to rural township and community hospitals, village clinics, and various technical agencies for specific disease prevention and control.

However, China' disease prevention and control development encountered difficulties during this period. Due to insufficient government inputs and breakup of the three-tiered medical and preventive healthcare network in rural area, from the mid-1980s, preventive services and immunization programs were allowed to charge fees, in order to fill the financial gaps and provide financial incentives to rural doctors to conduct vaccination work.

(4) Institutional Reform (1997–2003)

With social economic development, population aging, and changes in disease patterns, China's system on disease prevention and control could no longer meet the needs of the society and the wide population. In 1997, Shanghai consolidated the varied technical institutions into Shanghai Center for Disease Control and Prevention and Shanghai Health Inspection Center. This marked the beginning of comprehensive reforms in China's disease prevention and control system.

Based on the "Decisions by China's Central Committee of the Communist Party and the State Council on Healthcare Reform and Development," and the "Guidelines on Urban Healthcare Reform," and the reform progress of the disease prevention and control institutions across China, in April 2001, the Ministry of Health issued its "Guidelines on the Reform of the Disease Prevention and Control System," outlining the goals of the reform as well as the organizational structure. On Jan 23, 2002, Chinese Center for Disease Control and Prevention (China CDC), reorganized after the previous Chinese Academy of Preventive Medicine, was launched at the People's Great Hall. China Center for Health Inspection was also set up at the same time. The restructuring of Epidemic Prevention Stations into Centers for Disease Prevention and Control marked the beginning of China's new system of disease prevention and control. Figure 2.3 illustrates the components of China's public health system, which comprises health administrations at various levels, hospitals, disease prevention and control institutions, and health monitoring and supervision institutions.

(5) Rapid Development After 2003

Since the outbreak of SARS in 2003, the government has striven to put in place a comprehensive, coordinated, and sustainable scientific development concept, with a greater emphasis on "the people's well-being" and "community management" aiming to build a harmonious socialist society. Health and healthcare services are an area that all citizens are concerned with and a key enterprise that

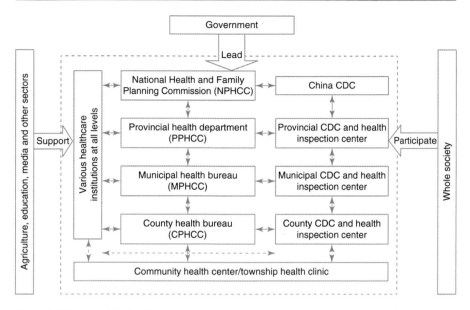

Fig. 2.3 China's public health system

has a profound bearing on the overall situation in China. It is also an area that involves the matter of social justice, which requires public policy for its realization and assurance.

As governance concepts and public policy paradigms changed, the healthcare reform in China became more comprehensive with increasingly clear goals being established. At the Third Plenary Session of the 16th CPC Central Committee in 2003, the concept of "deepening reform in public health" was proposed, while at the Fifth Plenary Session of the 16th CPC Central Committee in 2005, it was advocated that China works to "enhance the state of health of the people, increase government investment in health services, and make further improvements to the healthcare system." In 2006, at the 6th Plenary Session of the 16th CPC Central Committee, the official line was that China was to "remain committed to the public- welfare nature of public healthcare and health services, deepen reform in the healthcare system, enhance government responsibilities, undertake strict supervision and management, establish a basic health system that covers both urban and rural residents, and provide safe, effective, convenient, and cheap public health and basic medical services for the people." In 2007, the 17th CPC National Congress proposed "universal coverage of essential medical and healthcare services" as one new requirement to achieve the goal of building a "moderately prosperous society in an all-round way" and specified "the establishment of an essential healthcare system to enhance the state of health of all citizens," "the establishment of a public health service system, medical service system, health insurance system, and medicine supply assurance system that cover both urban and rural residents in order to provide safe, effective, convenient and affordable healthcare and health services for all." At the same time, a number of universities and research institutes conducted parallel studies on the national plan for healthcare reform. The results of these studies provided the basis for the *Opinions on the Deepening of Healthcare System Reform* issued by the CPC Central Committee and the State Council in April 2009. This document stated for the first time the goal of "equitable access to basic public health services." A series of initiatives were launched in the areas of funding, service standards, service content, etc. These initiatives have been implemented at the local level. Incremental progress has been achieved with increased primary public health workforce, strengthened capacity building to implement public health programs, strengthened institutional building, improved public health service delivery system, coordinated and cooperated working mechanism explored, public health functions effectively implemented, and accelerated development of the health information system for a timely and effective dissemination of public health information. While working on basic public health service programs, local governments with the concept of "the integration of prevention and treatment" explored new approach of government purchasing public health services and new models of health management and looked for solutions to improve regulation and assessment, to improve the precise management skills.

With the public health reform, China's basic public health services, both community-based and individual-based, have been delivered in a comprehensive way. The major public health programs have been implemented effectively, covering broad range of beneficiaries. The effectiveness of public health services continuously improves, and people's access to public health services is also becoming more equitable.

2.2.4   Public Health Achievements and Contributions in New China

(1) Public Health Service System

Public health practices require organized efforts from the society. Hence, looking at the various categories of organizations and institutions related to public health within a certain country will inform us more about the setup of the country's public health service system. Generally the system includes:

- National or local government agencies for public health. These agencies represent the government in providing public health services and also serve to provide support where necessary. These agencies include health, human resources and social security, land and resources, environmental protection, and planning and development authorities.
- International organizations for public health. China participates in the activities of such organizations by means of signed agreements, conventions. The organization is responsible for directing, supervising, and coordinating public health work in various countries and regions. Examples of such organizations include the World Health Organization (WHO), the International Red Cross (IRC), the

International Atomic Energy Agency (IAEA), and the United Nations Children's Fund (UNICEF).

- Healthcare providers, such as hospitals, community health service centers, mental health organizations, health check-up centers, and nursing homes, which mainly provide prevention, diagnostic, and care services.
- Agencies that support public health program implementation and related professional organizations, including police bureaus, fire departments, and emergency medical care centers managed by the government. Their main role is to prevent and handle emergencies and public health events.
- Environmental protection, labor protection, and food safety agencies. These are law enforcement agencies responsible for monitoring the living environment and making sure that it remains safe for the sake of the population's health. Cultural, education, and sports organizations work on the neighborhood level to provide the spiritual and material environment for health promotion.
- Health-related nongovernment organizations in the field. These organizations provide policy and material support to disadvantaged communities, including the physically and mentally disadvantaged, low-income persons, persons living alone, and the elderly.

China's public health service system is made up of two functional components: a professional public health services network and a medical service network. The professional public health services network is in turn made up of professional public health institutions working in the following areas: disease prevention and control, health education, maternal and child health, mental health services, emergency treatment, the collection and supply of blood, health monitoring and supervision, and family planning. Currently, China's basic public health service programs are mainly delivered free of charge to all citizens through village and township health centers, village clinics, and neighborhood community health service centers and stations in urban areas, with other community healthcare organizations serving to complement such services. Major public health service programs are mainly delivered through professional public health institutions. In accordance with the law, hospitals are responsible for monitoring, reporting, and handling major illnesses and public health emergencies as well as other public health services as stipulated by the state.

The document of *Opinions on Deepening of Healthcare Reform* released by the CPC Central Committee and the State Council called for the comprehensive enhancement of China's public health service system. The two organs called for the establishment and building-up of a professional public health service network in the areas of disease prevention and control, health education, the provision of maternal and child healthcare, the provision of mental health services, the provision of emergency treatment, the collection and supply of blood, health monitoring and supervision, family planning, etc. The two also called for further improvement of the public health service functions of the medical service system which is based on the community health service network. The public health service system should be established with clear responsibilities, information exchange, resource-sharing, and high levels of coordination, aiming to enhance the system's capacity of service delivery and public health emergency response, leading to a more equitable access to the basic public health services in both urban and rural areas.

After decades' efforts, the number of health professionals per 1000 people rose from 0.93 in 1949 to 4.15 in 2009, while the number of beds in healthcare facilities per 1000 people grew from 0.18 in 1950 to 3.8 in 2011. By 2011, there were a total of 37,000 township hospitals in 33,000 townships, 660,000 village clinics in 590,000 administrative villages, 7776 community health centers, and 25,000 community health stations in 7110 communities. There were also 1.53 village health workers per 1000 rural residents. The statistics have shown remarkable improvements in the accessibility of healthcare services, especially in rural China.

(2) Public Health Legislation

Over the last six decades, China has made significant achievements in the area of health legislation. A total of 10 laws have been passed and promulgated by the National People's Congress, with 27 regulations approved and/or put out by the State Council. In addition, the National Health and Family Planning Commission (formerly the Ministry of Health) has also put in place over 400 regulations and nearly 2000 health standards. In 2009, the CPC Central Committee and the State Council also stated in the *Opinions on Deepening of Healthcare Reform* that efforts should be made to improve the health legislation and speed up the legislation for basic health services and gradually establish a comprehensive legal framework for health development in line with China's basic medical and healthcare system. In the next few years, China will make great efforts to strengthen its health legislation, especially to establish the Basic Health Law, the fundamental law to guide China's overall health development; this important law is expected to be approved in recent years.

As of 2012, the laws related to disease prevention and control that have been implemented include the Food Safety Law (2009), the Law on Prevention and Control of Infectious Diseases (2004), the Population and Family Planning Law (2001), the Prevention and Control of Occupational Diseases Law (2001), the Drug Administration Law (2001), the Law on Practicing Doctors (1998), the Blood Donation Law (1997), the Maternal and Infant Healthcare Law (1994), the Law of the People's Republic of China on the Red Cross Society (1993), and the Frontier Health and Quarantine Law (1986). In addition, the Food Hygiene Law of 1995 was superseded with the promulgation of the Food Safety Law in 2009.

As of 2012, the administrative regulations related to disease prevention and control which are implemented are the following:

- Special Rules on the Labor Protection of Female Employees (2012)
- Management Approaches for Depositories of Pathogenic Microbial Bacteria (Toxins) Species that Cause Infections in Humans (2009)
- Management Approaches (Trial) for Urban Community Health Service Agencies (2006)
- Regulations for the Prevention and Treatment of Schistosomiasis (2006)
- Management Regulations for the Transport of Highly Pathogenic Microbial Bacteria (Toxins) Species or Samples Capable of Infecting Humans (2005)

- The People's Republic of China Approaches to Frontier Health Monitoring and Supervision (1982) Regulations on the Management of Narcotic Drugs and Psychotropic Drugs (2005)
- Regulations on the Protection of Chinese Medicines (1993)
- Regulations on the Management of Family Planning Efforts for Migrant Populations (1999)
- Regulations on Health Quarantine on Domestic Transport (1999)
- Management Regulations on the Supervision of Medical Equipment (2000)
- The People's Republic of China Ordinances on Chinese Medicine (2003)
- The People's Republic of China
- Regulations on the Implementation of the Drug Administration Law (2002)
- Regulations on Responses to Public Health Emergencies (2003)
- Regulations on the Management of Medical Waste (2003)
- Regulations on the Management of Rural Medical Practitioners (2003)
- Management Regulations for the Biosecurity of Pathogenic Microbiology Laboratories (2004) Regulations on the Management of Healthcare Institutions (1994)
- The People's Republic of China Regulations on the Use of the Red Cross Logo (1996)
- The People's Republic of China Implementation Measures for the Maternal and Infant Healthcare Law (2001)
- Regulations on Family Planning Technical Services (2001)
- Regulations on the Management of Healthcare Malpractice (2002)
- Labor Protection Regulations for the Use of Toxic Substances in the Workplace (2002)
- The People's Republic of China Regulations on the Prevention and Treatment of Pneumoconiosis (1987) Several Provisions on the Monitoring and Management of Acquired Immunodeficiency Disease (1988) Approaches for the Management of Toxic Drugs Used in Healthcare (1988)
- Approaches for the Management of Radiopharmaceuticals (1989)
- The People's Republic of China Implementation Rules for the Frontier Health Inspection and Quarantine Law (1989)
- Regulations for Protection Against Radioactive Isotopes and Radiation Devices (1989)
- Regulations for the Health Monitoring and Supervision of Cosmetic Products (1990)
- Regulations on School Health (1990)
- The People's Republic of China Implementation Rules for the Prevention and Control of Infectious Diseases Law (1991)
- Regulations on the Iodization of Edible Salt for the Elimination of Iodine Deficiency (1994)
- Regulations on the Management of Blood Products (1996)
- Regulations on the Management of Sanitation in Public Places (1987)

In addition, administration regulations that have been abolished include the Regulations on the Labor Protection of Female Officers (established 1988) in favor of the Special Regulations on the Labor Protection of Female Officers (instituted

2012), the Regulations on the Management of Psychotropic Drugs (e. 1988) and the Regulations on the Management of Narcotic Drugs (e. 1987) in favor of the Regulations on the Management of Narcotic and Psychotropic Drugs (e. 2005), and the Regulations for Radiation Protection Against Radioactive Isotopes and Radiation Equipment.

(3) Human Resource Development in Public Health

Health workforce is an important component of a nation (and region)'s health system. It plays crucial role to maintain and strengthen its own health system functions, and it is the basic element of health resource [9]. According to WHO, "the health workforce consists of all people engaged in actions whose primary intent is to improve health. This includes health service providers, such as doctors, nurses, midwives, pharmacists and community health officers. It also includes health management and support officers, such as hospital administrators, district health managers and social officers, who dedicate all or part of their time to improving health."

China defines health human resource as those who are employed in health institutions for medical services, public health, medical research, and on-the-job education, including health professionals, village doctors and rural health workers, other technical staff, administration and management, and logistic staff. Here, "health professionals" refer to practicing physicians and assistant physicians, registered nurses, pharmacists, technicians, etc. "Village doctors and rural health workers" are those who have obtained rural healthcare licenses and who are engaged in the work of disease prevention, healthcare, and general medical services in rural healthcare institutions. The term "rural health workers" refers to those working in rural healthcare facilities and who do not hold the requisite licensing to serve as rural physicians. "Other technical staffs" are individuals who work in healthcare institutions and who are engaged in nonmedical jobs such as equipment maintainance, health communication, information technology, and research and teaching. "Administration and management" are individuals who manage the health facilities' operation on the technical areas such as medical services, public health, medical research and teaching, and the administrative tasks such as party administration, human resources, finance, information management, safety and security, etc. "Logistic staff" are those who conduct equipment operation and maintenance, logistic support, and service in health facilities, and these logistic staffs can be classified into technical and nontechnical— with the formal including nursing workers, pharmacy staff, inspectors, cashiers, patient registration staff, etc.

By the end of 2013, the number of health workforce in China amounts to 9.79 million, including 7.211 million health professionals, 1.081 million village doctors and rural health workers, 360,000 other technical staffs, 421,000 in administration and management, and 718,000 logistic staffs. Among health professionals, there were 2.795 million practicing physicians and assistant physicians (including 146,000 general practitioners) and 2.783 million registered nurses. By the end of

2013, the distribution of health professionals was as follows: 5.371 million (54.9% of the total) employed in hospitals, 3.514 million (35.9%) in community healthcare institutions, and 826,000 (8.4%) in professional public health institutions. In 2013, there were 2.06 practicing (assistant) physicians and 2.05 registered nurses per 1000 people, 1.07 general practitioners, and 6.08 public health professionals per 10,000 population.

Global statistics indicates that the average density of doctors per 10,000 population is 17, while that of nurses is 28; in China the density of health workforce, especially the nurses, is lower than the world average, and that of the physicians is lower than the mid- and high-income countries. The annual average growth rate (4.6%) of health workforce, compared with the speed of GDP growth and health service demand, is far lagging behind.

In China, public health professionals work in the areas of disease prevention and control, health education and health promotion, occupational health, environmental health, nutrition and food safety, radiation safety, and school health, emergency management, maternal and child health, emergency medicine, the collection and supply of blood, and mental health services, as well as technical staff working in public health. Professionals working in the national, provincial, city, and county public health institutions are China's main public health workforce. Generally speaking, China's public health workforce is insufficient in quantities, and the technical capacities need to be strengthened. There are only 1.4 disease prevention and control personnel in place for every 10,000 population in China, which is one-fifth of the ratio in the USA. Human resources are especially lacking in the areas of food safety, health education, maternal and child health, and the collection and supply of blood. Health emergency workforce, in huge demand of management and technical expertise, is scattered in health authorities, supervision agencies, universities, and research institutions, requiring great efforts to consolidate. There is a serious lack of professionals working in medical emergency care, especially physicians, for whom huge disparities exist between big cities and the central/western region; and one prehospital emergency personnel serve a total population of 126,000, which is a huge gap compared with that of international data − 10,000. In 2009, China's mental health institutions employed 64,000 health workers, only 0.9% of whom are mental health physicians; the demand for mental health professionals is huge. The same workforce shortage can be observed in the area of blood collection and supply, with low education qualification and small number of young professionals, particularly in need of the blood transfusion technicians and blood transfusion physicians.

(4) Public Health Surveillance and Information System

In the 1950s, the US CDC applied surveillance and monitoring systems into the area of public health. In the 1970s, the concept of disease surveillance was introduced to China. Up to the present, China has preliminarily established the disease surveillance system that covers various key health issues and high-risk population throughout all life course. The development of China's disease surveillance system reflects the history of China's public health development over the last six decades. Between 1950 and 1980, the focus was on the mandatory reporting of notifiable infectious diseases, and efforts began to establish surveillance of specific key infectious diseases (such as influenza and hemorrhagic fever); the tumor registration system was also established in this period. Between 1980 and 2000, new concepts and methods of surveillance were introduced to China, and a comprehensive disease surveillance system was established. The new system was used to monitor elements such as congenital defects, cause of death, chronic diseases, and behavioral risk factors. Since 2000, online direct reporting system has been enforced for notifiable infectious diseases, together with emergency surveillance and early warning mechanism for epidemic outbreaks.

Health surveillance systems in China fall into three categories in terms of targets of surveillance: surveillance systems for infectious diseases; surveillance systems for chronic, noninfectious diseases and related risk factors; and surveillance systems for other key health issues.

First, the surveillance of infectious diseases is based mainly on the mandatory reporting of notifiable infectious diseases and supplemented by various other single-disease surveillance system. Surveillance is conducted based on the level of prevention and control required. Key infectious diseases under surveillance include tuberculosis, AIDS, Hepatitis B, and schistosomiasis. There are another 26 "focus diseases" under surveillance, including plague and cholera. Active and passive surveillance is conducted both through laboratory surveillance and population surveillance. In the future, laboratory capabilities (such as in the areas of serology and etiology) will be further enhanced, together with the necessary forecasting and early warning capabilities and the capability to discover emerging infectious diseases early.

Second, compared to the surveillance of infectious diseases, surveillance of chronic diseases and related risk factors started in China late, and the relevant systems and methods are still being refined. Currently, the surveillance systems that are already in place include tumor registration, tracking of cause of death, surveys of risk factors for chronic diseases, and the surveillance of key diseases (cardiovascular and cerebrovascular diseases); however, chronic diseases like cardiovascular and cerebrovascular diseases and cancers have already become the major public health issues threatening the health of Chinese residents, while China's chronic disease surveillance capabilities cannot meet the need of disease prevention and control challenges, with still a long way to go.

Third, among other health-related surveillance systems, including birth-defect monitoring, food safety-risk monitoring, and reports of public health issues such as chemical contaminants and harmful factors in food, foodborne pathogens, foodborne diseases, public health emergencies, etc., the public health emergency reporting mechanism is the one with Chinese characteristics. The mechanism deploys various types of reports (11 types of incidents) and level-specific responses (at four different levels). Apart from the aforementioned surveillance systems, new surveillance systems are also constantly emerging in various regions or introduced by various institutions, such as the monitoring of antibiotic resistance and hospital-acquired infections; new surveillance technologies are also being deployed, such as symptom monitoring and public opinion monitoring technologies.

Generally speaking, China's disease surveillance system is constantly improving, with the surveillance contents in expansion and methods further reformed.

(5) Disease Prevention and Control

Public health functions fulfilled by China's facilities on disease prevention and control are expanding. According to a report, China's public health functions can be divided into 25 categories which include 78 items covering 255 specific programs. The 25 categories cover such areas as disease control, emergency response, surveillance and information, risk factor intervention, experimental testing, health education and promotion, technical guidance and applied studies, etc.; the functions of the disease prevention and control agencies at the community level cover information collection, planned immunization, the prevention and control of infectious diseases, the prevention and control of tuberculosis, the prevention and control of AIDS, the prevention and control of parasites and local diseases, disinfection, health education, school health, the prevention and control of chronic diseases, risk factor intervention, the prevention and control of mental illness, and emergency handling, altogether 13 items. China's public health has made remarkable progress from different perspectives—the functions and services, the development, and the need; however, there is a huge gap before achieving the goal of universal health coverage for all.

Immunization is an effective strategy to prevent, control, and even eradicate infectious diseases. China was one of the earliest countries to prevent infectious disease by means of artificial immunization. After the founding of People's Republic of China in 1949, the government attached great importance to the health of the children, as well as the prevention and healthcare work; therefore, China's immunization program expanded rapidly and progressed through three phases in its development: emergency immunization, planned immunization, and national program on immunization.

In 1974, the 27th World Health Assembly passed a resolution to "develop and adhere to the immunization method and the monitoring plan for infectious diseases in order to prevent and control infectious diseases such as smallpox, diphtheria, poliomyelitis, pertussis, tetanus, tuberculosis." This resolution was approved in the context of the global eradiation of smallpox, and in developing countries (not including China), infectious diseases were proved to be preventable by vaccines, while in developed countries, infectious diseases for children have been successfully controlled. The resolution marked the official launch of the Expanded Program on Immunization (EPI) worldwide. EPI covers two parts: one is to expand the coverage of immunization population and to increase the immunization rate; the other is to promote the usage of safe, effective, and new vaccines and expand the types of vaccines. Based on its particular requirements, China introduced the concept of planned immunization with children as the target service population. The planned immunization developed rapidly in China. Developments in this area can be divided into three phases: the first phase between 1978 and 1984 saw an emphasis on developing the basic planned immunization program; the second period (1985–1990) saw a push by provincial and county units to achieve an immunization rate of

85%; and in the third phase (1991–2000), efforts were focused on maintaining the immunization rate and the control and eradication of targeted infectious diseases. The characteristics of China's planned immunization phase are as follows:

- The immunization approach shifted significantly to a more comprehensive one, with strategies such as routine immunization, targeted immunization, and emergency immunization.
- Coverage has continued to grow, with new vaccines for Hepatitis B, epidemic meningitis, Japanese encephalitis, measles/mumps/rubella, and Hepatitis A adding to the existing battery of the "four basic vaccines."
- The schedule for the national child immunization program was established.
- The system of immunization service has been further enhanced.
- Legislative support has been established for the task of immunization, which has also entered a period of standardized management.
- A planned immunization cold-chain system, which provides more than six immunization services a year to regions home to more than 90% of China's population, has more or less been established.
- China has embarked on a large number of partnerships with international partners which have yielded much positive results.
- China has realized the goal of universal child immunization as tabled by the WHO.
- China has also made significant progress in terms of the monitoring of the impact of immunization on infectious disease incidence rates.
- Decisive advancements have been made in efforts to eradicate polio, and incidence rates for infectious diseases covered by the immunization program are at a historic low.

In 2001, the national program on immunization started, and the government implemented its national expanded program on immunization in 2007. The overall objectives were to fully implement the expanded program on immunization, keep China polio-free, eradicate measles, have Hepatitis B under control, and further reduce the incidence rate of infectious diseases that can be prevented by vaccination. Four evaluation indicators were raised:

- Immunization against Hepatitis B, tuberculosis (in the form of the BCG vaccine),"DTP"(diphtheria, tetanus, and pertussis), and measles in children of the appropriate age levels should be at least 90% at the county level by the year 2010.
- Children of the appropriate age across the country should be immunized against epidemic meningitis, Japanese encephalitis, and Hepatitis A by the year 2010.
- The immunization rate for the target population of the hemorrhagic fever vaccine should be at least 70%. Fourth, the immunization rate for the target population of the anthrax and leptospirosis vaccines should be at least 70%.

After a few decades of hard work, China's immunization program has yielded impressive achievements. The government has consistently increased its funding for the program and established a professional, dedicated team in the area on a nationwide basis. A complete cold-chain system has been established, and legislative support is created for the task of immunization planning. During the period of standardized management, the incidence of targeted infectious diseases declined significantly. A good number of partnerships established with international partners have resulted in strong outcomes, while China has also made impressive achievements in the establishment of its surveillance network. The number of diseases included in the national immunization program is constantly growing. In particular, China has made significant advances in its efforts upon eradicating polio and measles and controlling Hepatitis B. This has significantly contributed to the prevention and control of diseases.

(6) Health Education and Health Promotion

In the 1950s and 1960s, China's health education was conducted through "patriotic health campaign." Health education efforts were disrupted for a period of time due to the Cultural Revolution and were soon recovered after the economic reform in late 1970s. In 1984, the China Association of Health Education was established, followed by the China Health Education Institute (now the China Health Education Center) in 1986. The provincial and city health education centers also resumed to function. By late 1980s, there were a total of 26 provincial-level health education centers and over 150 centers at the city level with nearly 20,000 persons employed in health education.

China began to train health education professionals in the early 1980s. In 1984, the then-Hebei Medical College became the first school to offer a program on health education, and its first cohort of students in 1985 consisted of high-school graduates who could receive full-time training in the college. Completion of the program resulted in a 3 years' degree. Subsequently, Shanghai Medical University, Tongji Medical University, and Beijing Medical University all set up health education department to recruit students. Later on, the Anhui Medical University, Tongji Medical University, and certain vocational schools commenced professional and vocational programs in health education. Nearly 2000 health education professionals were trained at various institutions.

The *Chinese Journal of Health Education* was founded in 1985. The Journal is, to date, the only national-level professional and academic journal in the area of health education. In 1988, China published for the first time *Health Education*, edited by Jia Weilian et al. In 1989, the Shanghai Medical University published a translation of *The Precede-Proceed Model of Health Program Planning & Evaluation* written by famed health education expert Lawrence Green et al. This has had a significant impact on the promotion of theoretical studies and practice in health education in China.

Since the 1980s, health education practice has been mostly program-based, programs supported by the WHO and UNICEF in the mid-1980s, and later the self-funded health education program, as well as the health education practices within comprehensive health programs. Currently, a variety of technical areas such as tobacco control, the prevention and control of AIDS, the prevention and control of tuberculosis, the prevention and control of chronic disease (hypertension), and maternal and child health have been integrated into the routine work of health education and health promotion, with the corresponding evaluation indicators established. In addition, integrated health education programs have been conducted in schools, workplaces, hospitals, and communities through the setting-based health-promoting programs, such as "health-promoting schools," health-promoting hospitals," "healthy villages," and "healthy cities."

When we look back on the evolution of China's health education, it seemed that China's health education is mostly focused on the practical efforts to solve the actual health problems, less on the research and theoretical studies. But we can always discover the theories behind the practices.

First, the dissemination of health knowledge has been an important part of health education work, from the case of Ding County to other areas in the 1930s. The focus of health knowledge dissemination is to bring health knowledge to the general population through the approach of publicity. In particular during the 1950s and 1960s, wide publicity activities were conducted to raise public awareness on basic health information and knowledge.

In terms of the essence of publicity, the expected outcome was public awareness, and the methods used included lectures, newspaper columns, slogans, and radio. This kind of information dissemination method is basically one-way communication, with insufficient information feedback and lack of attention leading to actual behavioral change. However, given the historical context where there was only one source of information and the people's value orientation was also relatively simpler, and that the focus of intervention was on environmental health and personal hygiene, even one-way communication was useful in triggering change in the behavior of the general public, who were especially proactive in participating in environmental cleanup and other organized efforts.

China's approach to disseminate health knowledge is quite different from the health education concept in other countries. Their concept is to empower the people with knowledge and skills so that they could change the behavior and lifestyles voluntarily, and this change is from the raised personal awareness, while China's approach is a combination of offering knowledge and reinforcing government leadership and community mobilization [10]. Behavioral change was seen as due to both enhancement of the individual's knowledge as well as the result of social and cultural influence. To a very large extent, this model has made up for the inadequacies in the impact of a pure publicity campaign on individual behavior.

Second, health education. In the mid-1980s, modern pedagogy of health education was introduced to China, and approaches such as specialization were taken in order to cultivate health education professionals. The establishment of a national-level health education institution, the China Health Education Center, and a growing number of international exchanges all played a role in promoting the development of health education theory in China and also helped those in the fields of health education and health promotion to become better aligned with theories in the international arena.

Health education is based on the theory of psychological behavior, to study how people's health-related behaviors are formed and changed. The focus is on the causes of such change at the individual level and to identify individual factors—like knowledge, beliefs, attitudes, and capabilities—that play a role in behavioral change [11]. As we know, "education" plays an important role in the enhancement of health knowledge, the establishment of healthy values and attitudes, and the enhancement of the individual's ability to accept healthy behaviors. Furthermore, "education" is even more focused on the process of internal change in the "subject of education." Hence, the concept of health education proposed has underscored the value of education in behavioral change as well as the individual's willingness to change his or her behavior.

The aforementioned concept emphasizes the idea that the core of health education is to influence the individual or group to refrain from unhealthy behaviors and ways of life. It is believed that in order to realize behavioral change, the individual or the group must first be in possession of health-related knowledge, enhance knowledge levels, and establish the desire to pursue health and health-centered values. The individual then makes the decision to make behavioral changes with information in hand and knowledge levels enhanced. In addition, this concept also highlights information dissemination and behavioral intervention as the main means of educating the individual.

In terms of theoretical research, the contributions of domestic scholars and health education professionals can be categorized into two areas. (1) They have tested western theories on health education and health-related behavior in the Chinese cultural context, such as by designing tests of various health education methods in specific regions, the effectiveness of intervention with specific health-related behaviors, the expression of theories of health communication in practice, the use of the Health Belief model and Stages of Change theories in areas such as the drug compliance of hypertensive patients, and behavioral intervention with smokers and diabetes patients. (2) They have, based on health education theories, provided national and local administrations with technical support and the basis for decision-making in the areas of health education development and the development of mass health services. Examples of such support include providing national and local health planners with information for planning purposes, as well as for state-level health development programs.

Third, health promotion. In China, the concept of health promotion was introduced around the same time as the idea of health education was introduced, that is, in the mid-1980s. Therefore, it is difficult to separate these two concepts in terms of theoretical studies and practice. From the disciplinary perspective, the majority of domestic academics recognize health education as an independent discipline with its own theoretical system, while health promotion is more widely regarded as a form of public health strategy rather than a stand-alone discipline. In the mid-1990s, the World Bank granted a loan project "Health VII." Although the content of the program was not limited to health promotion, it pioneered the practice of risk factor monitoring in China. The program, which was also the first to use "health promotion" as its program title, focused on intervention, specifically with salt intake and physical exercise with regard to cardiovascular diseases. Health promotion school program launched at the same time had a better explanation of the contents of health promotion, which has integrated health policy, environmental support, and school health education into one package for the promotion of student health.

China is a large country, and the health issues form a complex array at various levels. The population is threatened by old and new infectious diseases, and in some places, maternal and child health and nutrition are still big health problems. At the same time, there are also the pressures caused by the aging of large numbers of people and chronic diseases. In the last 30 years, theoretical developments in the area of the health promotion in China have mostly to do with how to apply core concepts into the specific circumstances, such as developing hygienic cities, healthy cities, tobacco control, the prevention and control of AIDS and tuberculosis, as well as establishing comprehensive chronic disease prevention and control demonstration zones.

(7) Patriotic Health Campaign

Patriotic health campaign was launched right after the founding of the People's Republic of China in 1949, to address the urban and rural environmental cleanliness and combat the epidemics of infectious diseases that were left by the war and old society. Party organizations and governments at different levels began to launch mass health campaigns. The Government Administration Council (GAC) established the Central Epidemic Prevention Committee in October 1949 due to an outbreak of plague in Chabei district (Northwest Hebei today). In 1952, during the Korean War, the US army used biological weapons, dropping insects, and rodents carrying pathogenic microorganisms in North Korea and border areas of China. In response, in March 1952 the GAC decided to revive the Central Epidemic Prevention Committee. In December of the same year, the committee was renamed the Central Patriotic Health Campaign Committee, with its first head then-Premier Zhou Enlai. In accordance with the requirements from the central government, Patriotic Health Campaign Committees were established at various levels, across different sectors and in all workplaces. These Committees organized residents in both rural and urban areas and staff in workplaces to conduct environmental cleanups, as well as the extermination of disease-carrying pests such as houseflies, mosquitoes, fleas, and rats. Chairman Mao also gave inspiring calling to this movement: "Mobilize everybody to pay attention to personal hygiene, to reduce diseases and improve people's health, to smash the enemy's bacteriological warfare to pieces." Subsequently, patriotic health campaigns went into full swing across the country. In August 1998, the State Council decided to rename the Patriotic Health Campaign Committee to the National Patriotic Health Campaign Committee.

The specific context in which the Committee (and its work) emerged means that its name bears strong political connotations. The use of the word "patriotic" in the name of the Committee required the people to place the work of the corresponding health-related efforts on the same level of importance of the nation itself, while the term "health" described the scope of such efforts, and the term "campaign" specified the means of social mobilization.

Following victory in the Korean War, the central Party apparatus and the State Council continued to focus on patriotic health campaigns as a main approach in health-related efforts. Such campaigns have yielded rich results over various historical periods, helping to promote health, change behaviors, and reform the country. In the 1950s and 1960s, patriotic health campaign activities were vigorously conducted nationwide. People were asked to improve the environmental appearance, eradicate the "four pests," and raise awareness of basic health knowledge. The response from Chinese society and the masses was overwhelmingly positive, and significant achievements were made. The campaign was affected by the Cultural Revolution (1966–1976). In 1978, after the Cultural Revolution ended, the State Council re-established the Central Patriotic Health Campaign Committee and issued the *Notification on Continuing Patriotic Health Campaign*. At a National Patriotic Health Campaign Conference held in Yantai of Shandong province, the Central Patriotic Health Campaign Committee specified its priority work as improving urban cities' environmental health and managing water and sewage in the rural areas, and the root causes also need to be addressed. Local Party Committees and local governments responded to the central government's request positively and quickly restored the management offices with their organizational network; therefore, actions to improve environmental cleanliness, drinking water management, and waste management of human and animal wastes were taken passionately again by the whole society across China.

The State Council's *Decision to Strengthen Patriotic Health Work* issued in 1989 marked the beginning of a new phase for patriotic health campaigns in China. The Decision emphasized once again that using "the population-based patriotic health approach to combat disease is a successful experience created by our nation." In the same document, the State Council called for further enhancement of patriotic health work in response to the challenges such as the negative environmental health due to rapid economic development, high incidence of some infectious diseases, and the low health awareness among the general public. The State Council asked the patriotic health campaign to be strengthened through the implementation of the priorities such as improving environmental health, rural water management, and health education for all.

According to the State Council's *Decision to Strengthen Patriotic Health Work*, aiming to upgrade the urban infrastructure and health management standards, from 1989 with the endorsement of the State Council, the National Patriotic Health Campaign Committee launched the initiative of National Hygiene City. Four major inspections were organized by the National Patriotic Health Campaign Committee nationwide in the 1990s. Subsequently, a batch of cities, districts, and towns were awarded "National Hygienic Cities," "National Hygienic Districts," and "National Hygienic Towns" through an application mechanism. At the same time, provinces, autonomous regions, and municipalities also conducted the provincial initiative with the same mechanism and approaches. Through these initiatives, the urban and rural environmental cleanliness have been improved, which contributed to a better working and living environment for the people. The National Patriotic Health Campaign Committee established standards and management regulations for cities, districts, and towns, in order to ensure that health inspection work in the cities would be carried out over the long term in a standardized manner toward a scientific and regular trend. Overall, the initiatives to developing hygienic cities/districts/counties have become a new platform for the patriotic health campaign work.

In February 2014, the State Council issued the *Opinions on Further Strengthening Patriotic Health Work in a New Era* ([2014] 66). This policy, an important guidance from the State Council on patriotic health campaign work over 25 years since 1989, puts forward specific requirements in the new social economic context. Premier Li Keqiang had important comment: "Patriotic health campaigns are irreplaceable in prevention and reduction of diseases, and in improving urban and rural environmental health, as well as in the enhancement of the civilization and health literacy for all. It is important for the government at all levels across all sectors to take actions on addressing the key heath concerns through implementing the patriotic health campaign activities with innovative approaches and with integrated efforts of health reform, along with the efforts to raise awareness on public health, to strengthen the development of patriotic health organizations and primary healthcare service system. Efforts should be made to control the sources and to address the root causes, to implement human-centered, population-based practices, to conduct cleanliness actions and promote the development of hygienic villages, communities and cities, to promote healthy lifestyle so as to reduce the incidence of diseases and the transmission, to contribute to the development of a healthy China and bring happiness to all Chinese population."

In the 1980s, countries in Europe and North America launched campaigns for the building of Healthy Cities and received strong responses from several nations and cities. Currently, Healthy City campaigns have been launched in 4500 cities worldwide. China's Ministry of Health cooperated with WHO in 1994 to launch Healthy City programs in Chaoyang District in Beijing, Jiading County in Shanghai, etc. A number of cities and districts also joined the program. In 2007, the Office of the National Patriotic Health Campaign Committee established Healthy City pilots in six cities (Shanghai, Hangzhou, Dalian, Suzhou, Zhangjiagang, and Karamay), two districts in Beijing, and two towns in Shanghai. At the same time, a number of Chinese cities also proactively made their own Healthy City efforts. Patriotic Health Campaign Committee at national and sub-national level implemented various health programs which enabled the traditional patriotic health work expanded to new areas and also upgraded the development of the existing hygienic cities.

Patriotic health campaign is one noteworthy characteristic of China's public health, adhering to the principles of social mobilization, community participation, and creation of a health promoting and maintaining environment. This is also the core concept for health promotion. The nationwide patriotic health campaign has made incredible contribution to the prevention of infectious intestinal diseases, parasitic disease, and zoonotic diseases by enabling a significant increase in the rates of safe drinking water and improved sanitation facilities. Statistics show that the available tap water in rural area rose from 68.4% in 2009 to 71.2% in 2010 while that of improved sanitation facilities has risen from 7.5% in 1993 to 72% in 2012. In addition, per capita housing area has also increased, which has facilitated the efforts toward the prevention of infectious respiratory diseases. Per capita housing area in China has risen from 3.6 m^2 in 1979 to 19 m^2 in 2000 and 27 m^2 in 2010.

(8) Improved Health Outcome

First, with the economic level of a low- and middle-income country, China has achieved the same health outcomes for its population as an upper-middle-income country. However, China is still in the primary stage of socialism; with its per capita income of USD 6890 (2009) which belongs to the category of low- and middle-income countries (USD 10,597, the same year), the health expenditure accounts for 4.3% of the total GDP, still a big gap compared with upper income countries (11.1%), while the density of doctors per 10,000 population is 14, much lower than that of the upper income countries (29 per 10,000). But even with constrained resources and huge population, China has achieved significant health improvement, with the average life expectancy at birth for male achieving 72 and for female 76, exceeding those of upper-middle-income countries (72 for males, 76 for females). China's infant mortality rate, mortality rate of children under 5 years, and maternal mortality rate are all at (or close to) the level of upper-middle-income countries.

Second, child health has made significant improvement. The maternal mortality rate and infant mortality rate are sensitive indicators to assess a country's health development [12]. In the past 60 years, China's maternal mortality rate has been on a linear decline, decreasing over 98% from 1500 per 100,000 at the early time of new China to 26.1 per 100,000 in 2011 (30.1 per 100,000 in rural areas). Similarly, the infant mortality rate has decreased dramatically, from 200‰ in 1949 to 12.1‰ in 2011 (16.1‰ in rural areas). In addition, the hospital delivery rate among Chinese women has increased from 43.7% in 1985 to 98.7% in 2011 and 96.7% in rural areas. The proportion of children below 5 years of age dying due to poor nutrition also decreased from 22% of total mortality in 2000 to 13% in 2010. The proportion of children under 5 with low body weight and who showed signs of delayed development also decreased significantly from 13.7% in 1990 to 3.6% in 2010 in the case of the former and from 33.1% in 1990 to 9.9% in 2010 in the case of the latter. The results of the fourth survey on the physical development of children released in 2006 show that on average, 6-year-old children were 6 cm taller and nearly 3 kg heavier than children of the same age 30 years ago. The national reported immunization rate has risen from 85% at the end of the last century to 95% of today. In summary, the data above shows that child health in China has seen significant improvements.

Third, infectious diseases have been effectively controlled. After six decades of unremitting efforts, outbreaks of infectious diseases in China have decreased in both frequency and scope, and the death rate has also been significantly lowered. The incidence rate for Class A and B infectious diseases has decreased from 7157.5 per 100,000 in 1970 to 238.8 per 100,000 in 2012; the mortality rate from Class A and B infectious diseases has also dropped from 56.0 per 100,000 in 1959 to 1.2 per 100,000 in 2012. Infectious disease is no longer the number one health killer in China, dropping to the eighth. The number of diseases that can be prevented by vaccines, insect-borne diseases, and infectious intestinal diseases has also declined significantly. China's last polio case occurred in 1994 (in 2000, Western Pacific Region). In 2006 the WHO announced that China was the first to eliminate filariasis. Smallpox was eradicated in 1961 in China (in 1978 in the world), and there have been significant achievements made in the control of biogeochemical and endemic diseases. China's infectious disease prevention and control cannot achieve such incredible outcomes without the hard work of public health professionals from generation to generation.

Fourth, prevention and control of chronic noncommunicable diseases have been strengthened. With socioeconomic development, China has entered into an aging society, with NCD becoming the key health threat for the Chinese population [13]. The last few decades saw remarkable progress in the prevention and control of NCDs in China. In the 1980s, the National Offices for the Prevention and Control of Tumors and Cerebrovascular Disease was established, strengthening efforts on tumors and cardiovascular diseases (CVD) prevention and control. In 1994, the Department of Epidemic Prevention in the Ministry of Health established an NCD office, with the implication of China's disease prevention and control shifting its focus from infectious diseases to NCDs. Two programs, one is World Bank's Health VII Project (health promotion program) in 1996, another one is Ministry of Health's community-based NCD prevention and control demonstration pilot in 1997, have strongly pushed forward China's NCD work. From 1998, community healthcare services have been widely conducted in the country, which became the "gatekeeper" of population health. In 2002, China CDC established NCD prevention and control center, aiming to strengthen the responsibilities of China CDC on addressing NCD challenges and also to enable CDC at all levels to play important roles in this regard; in the same year, the CVD prevention and control center of the Ministry of Health was established, aiming to strengthen CVD studies; in 2009, the National Cancer Center and the National Cardiovascular Disease Center were established with approval from the State Commission Office of Public Sectors Reform. Both centers were the first national-level institutions responsible for the integrated prevention and control of cancer and cardiovascular disease. Public health professionals in these professional institutions have made tremendous efforts to explore China's NCD prevention and control strategy. The past 20 years saw major changes in China's NCD strategy, which can be summarized into the following six aspects: from expert-led to government-led, from treatment-focused to prevention-focused, from tertiary hospital providing most services to primary healthcare taking over the responsibility, from urban areas to urban and rural areas, from health sector-led to all society's involvement, and from technical actions to community participation. China's NCD prevention and control system with the characteristics of community-based, social participation, government-led, rural areas with greater concern, and empowering individual skills is now on a good track to develop further.

At present, consensus has been reached on the goals, measures, priority population, and approaches of China's NCD work in the future. There are three goals: one is to improve peoples' healthy behavior; two is to conduct early diagnosis and early treatment; and three is to reduce incidence, reduce mortality, and reduce the rate of disability. The three priority groups of population cover the general population, high-risk population, and patients. There are three processes in NCD work: control of risk factors, early diagnosis and early treatment, and standardization of management. The three measures are being used: health education and health promotion, health management, and disease management. Four diseases should be given priority concerns: CVD, cancer, diabetes, and COPD. Four biological indicators—hypertension, hyperglycemia, dyslipidemia, and obesity together with four major risk factors including tobacco use, poor diet, insufficient exercise, and excessive alcohol intakes—should be given priorities for intervention.

Fifth, China has established the Health Insurance System, which includes the New Rural Cooperative Medicare Scheme, the Urban Employee Basic Medical Insurance, and the Urban Residents Basic Medical Insurance. The Health Insurance System is one of the most important achievements of China's Health Reform. By the end of 2011, over 95% of the population had joined one of the three insurances, with 800 million people enrolled in the New Rural Cooperative Medical Scheme. On average, 246 yuan per capita, including 210 from the government and 36 yuan from individual premium, was collected in the New Rural Cooperative Medical Scheme. In 2011, a total of 1.315 billion persons (times) benefited from the Basic Health Insurance System, with 70 million inpatients and 1 billion outpatients reimbursed [14]. At the same time, Rural Medical Assistance System was also established to subsidize the patients who cannot afford the medical expenses even after the reimbursement of the New Rural Cooperative Medical Scheme. A total population of 400 million has been covered by the Urban Employee Basic Medical Insurance and the Urban Residents Basic Medical Insurance. Rural migrant officers, informal employee, and officers in the enterprises with economic difficulties are all gradually integrated into the Basic Health Insurance System. Together with Medical Assistance System and all kinds of commercial insurances, China has achieved universal coverage of the health insurance for its people.

References

1. Crawford DH. Deadly companions: how microbes shaped our history. Oxford: Oxford University Press; 2007.
2. World Health Organization. Measurement of level of health. In: Technical reports series, vol. 137. Geneva: WHO; 1957.
3. Breslow L. A quantitative approach to the WHO definition of health: physical, mental and social wellbeing. Int J Epidemiol. 1972;1(4):347–55.
4. Berridge V. History in public health: a new development for history? Hygiea Int. 1999;1(1):23–35.
5. Li L. Challenges facing public health in China in the 21st century, and countermeasures. Chin J Health Educ. 2003;19(1):5–7.
6. Li L, Jiang Q. Theory and practice of public health in China. Beijing: People's Medical Publishing House; 2015.
7. Qingning Z, Susu L, Konglai Z. The establishment of Ting Hsien Experimental Project of Rural Health Service and its influence. Chin J Med Hist. 2016;46(4):221–8.
8. Zhiqian C. Chinese rural medicine. Chengdu: Sichuan People's Publishing House; 1998.
9. Li L. 60 years of public health in China: achievements and prospects. Chin J Public Health Manag. 2014;30(1):3–4.
10. Bangdiwala SI, Tucker JD, Zodpey S, et al. Public health education in India and China: history, opportunities, and challenges. Public Health Rev. 2011;33(1):204–24.
11. Green LW. Health education planning: a diagnostic approach. San Francisco: Mayfield Publishing Co; 1980.
12. Yu S. Focusing on prevention of key chronic diseases and risk factors. Shanghai J Prev Med. 2013;25(1):1–3, 10.
13. Li L. Reconsideration on 60 years of public health in China. Chin J Public Health Manag. 2014;30(3):311–5.
14. Jiahui S, Liming L. Hygiene and health: current situation and prospective. Chin J Prev Med. 2018;52(1):3–8.

Current Situation in China

3

Liming Li, Guangcai Duan, Haichao Lei, Xiaodong Tan, Chun Chang, and Weiyan Jian

3.1 Principles to Guide China's Health Development

In the past 60 years, the government's guiding principles to lead China's health work have changed over time. In August 1950, at the first National Health Conference jointly organized by the Ministry of Health and the Department of Health of the Central Military Commission, the guiding principle for health work was specified as "serving the workers, peasants and soldiers, prevention first, and integration of traditional Chinese medicine and Western medicine [1]." The second National Health Conference held in December 1952 reviewed the achievements and experience of germ wars and patriotic health campaigns, with Premier Zhou Enlai suggesting to add one more principle—"health work integrated with mass movement." Hence, the four core guiding principles for new China's health work were set up. The principle of "prevention first" provided clear direction on health development and requested every health professional to work hard not only to treat diseases for the people but also to combat diseases proactively through social mobilization. From 1950s to early 1960s, the effective implementation of the "prevention first" principle was one of the most important factors contributing to China's remarkable health achievements.

L. Li (✉) · C. Chang · W. Jian
School of Public Health, Peking University, Beijing, China
e-mail: lmlee@vip.163.com

G. Duan
School of Public Health, Zhengzhou University, Zhengzhou, China

H. Lei
Beijing Municipal Commission of Health and Family Planning, Beijing, China

X. Tan
School of Public Health, Wuhan University, Wuhan, Hubei, China

© Springer Nature Singapore Pte Ltd. and People's Medical Publishing House,
PR of China 2019
L. Li, Q. Jiang (eds.), *Introduction to Public Health in China*, Public Health in China,
https://doi.org/10.1007/978-981-13-6545-4_3

Over time, as the society developed, it became clear that the four principles established four decades ago had to be updated. On April 9, 1991, the 4th meeting of the 7th National People's Congress passed the *Outline of the Ten-Years Plan for National Economic and Social Development and the 8th Five-Year Plan*, specifying that China's health work should implement the principles of "prevention first, relying on science and technology advancement, social mobilization, integration of traditional Chinese medicine with Western medicine, and serving for people's health [2]." In the implementation process, the Ministry of Health put forward the strategic priorities: rural health, prevention care, and integration of traditional Chinese medicine and Western medicine for that period of time.

On January 15, 1997, the decision made by the CPC Central Committee and the State Council on the health reform and development set the guiding principles for the health work in the new era: "Rural health as the priority area, prevention first, integration of traditional Chinese medicine with Western medicine, relying on science, technology and education, social mobilization, and serving the people's health and serving the building of socialist modernization [3]." These principles, especially the last two of serving the people's health and serving the socialist modernization, were built upon understanding China's situation of "low level and wide coverage," which guided and promoted the sustained health development in China.

On August 19–20, 2016, China held its National Health Conference, which was the most important national meeting on health in 20 years. This important conference was held in the decisive stage of the country building a "moderately prosperous society." In an important speech, CPC Secretary General Xi Jinping underscored the importance of health development in the overall situation of the party and the government and provided insightful remarks on the significance, guiding principles, decisions, and arrangement of building healthy China, and he raised the urgent tasks and mission in order to ensure people's health, guiding us to continue exploring the way forward to develop Chinese health work with the basic adherence. His speech was a milestone in the history of China's health development. The conference specifically raised the new working principles: "focus on primary health care, driven by reform and innovation, prevention first, integration of traditional Chinese medicine and western medicine, health into all policies, co-building and sharing." "Focusing on primary health care" covers both rural and urban areas, comprehensively reflecting that primary health care is the health reform priority; "driven by reform and innovation" is the reflection of implementing the five development concepts of innovation, coordination, green, open, and sharing, while "prevention first, integration of traditional Chinese medicine and western medicine" follow the previous principles, reflecting health development and working principle with Chinese characteristics; "health in all policies" indicates the complex of health determinants and multi-sectoral cooperation, while "co-building and sharing" is the ultimate goal of China's health reform.

3.2 Health Service System

3.2.1 Health System

After the founding of new China in 1949, the government quickly developed its health system covering both urban and rural areas. Subsequently, China's health system has undergone a number of changes based on specific needs. In particular, the last two decades have seen constant adjustment and improvement in terms of financing, management, and service delivery.

Figure 3.1 shows the current structure of China's health system. Taxation income for the central and local governments constitutes public finance. One part of funding allocated to the health system from the public finance goes into the subsidizing of public health services institutions (CDCs, maternal and child health institutions, hospitals and community service institutions) through health administrations and other health-related government agencies. Public funding is also used to subsidize Urban and Rural Residents' Medical Insurance Program and Medical Assistance Program. Urban employees in formal sector pay premiums to the Urban Employee Basic Medical Insurance scheme. Chinese citizens are also free to purchase commercial medical insurances. When the insured makes use of health-care services, he or she may claim a part of expenses incurred from various medical insurance schemes. Various health facilities supported with the subsidization from public financing and (or) medical insurance provide medical services to Chinese people [4].

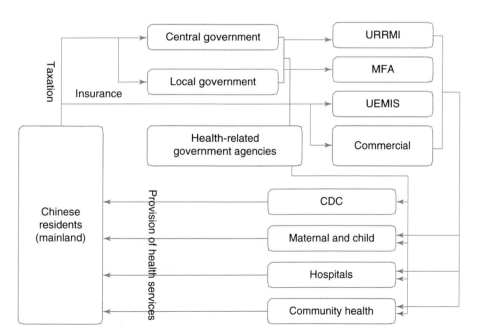

Fig. 3.1 China's health system

3.2.2   Health Service System

Like health service system in other countries, China's health service system provides its citizens with public health services and medical services. China's health service system comprises four types of health facilities at all levels (Fig. 3.2): CDCs, all hospitals, maternal and child health-care facilities, and community health service facilities (township hospital and village clinics in rural area). As of 2014, there were 3490 CDCs at various levels in China, as well as 3098 maternal and child health facilities, 25,860 hospitals, 34,238 community health services facilities, 36,902 township hospitals, and 645,470 village clinics. A total of 10,234,213 health officers were employed in the system, including 2,892,518 practicing physicians and assistant physicians and 3,004,144 registered nurses [5].

The CDCs provide public health services, including disease prevention and control, public health emergency response, information management of epidemic situation and health-related factors, the surveillance of health risk factors and interventions, laboratory testing and evaluation, health education and health promotion, etc. In addition, the CDCs also conduct technical trainings on disease prevention and control; provide technical guidance and technical support and services; undertake applied research; develop, introduce, and promote new technologies and methods; and guide the performance assessments.

The basic responsibilities of maternal and child health facilities at various levels are to provide public health services and basic medical services to women and children. The public health services include maternal and child health care; guide and conduct maternal and child health education and health promotion programs; and collect and analyze the data of maternal mortality, under-five mortality, and birth

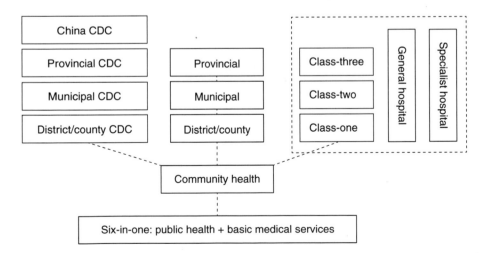

Fig. 3.2 Basic structure of China's health service system

defect surveillance. The basic medical services provided by maternal and child health facilities include diagnosis and treatment of common maternal and child diseases, family planning technical services, prenatal screening, health screening for newborns, and midwifery services; and based on specific needs and available resources, such services as prenatal diagnosis, the handling of obstetric complications, and emergency and critical treatment for newborns would be provided as well. In 2014, outpatient visits at maternal and child health facilities amounted to 230 million person (times) in China, with 8.703 million number of discharged patients [6].

Medical institutions provide clinical services. Clinical hospitals in China can be categorized into "general hospitals" and "specialist hospitals" according to the treated diseases. Depending on the size of the hospital, it may be classified as a tier-one, tier two, or tier-three hospital, with tier-three hospitals the largest. Theoretically, lower-level hospitals are supposed to treat patients with mild conditions, while more severe cases would be referred to higher-level hospitals. However, Chinese hospitals essentially provide both outpatient and hospitalization services; and under current policies, there was not a strict system of seeking community health service first as well as a referral system in place. Hospitals at various levels have duplicated functions with little coordination and cooperation. In 2014, there were a total of 2.97 billion outpatient visits at all levels across China, with the number of 150 million discharged patients.

Community health facilities provide primary health-care services to the community population and the families. The basic public health services include the management of resident health information; health education; the prevention and control of infectious diseases, endemic diseases, and parasitic diseases; the prevention and control of chronic diseases; mental health screening and community management; maternal and child health; health care for aging population; family planning counseling; and assisting public health emergency. These community health facilities also provide basic medical services, including the treatment of common diseases; nursing services and the treatment of patients with diagnosed chronic diseases; first-aid services; home-based medical services such as home visits, home care, and so on; referral services; and rehabilitation services. In 2014, a total of 690 million patient (times) visited community health facilities in Chinese cities, while a total of 3 billion patients were treated in township hospitals and village clinics in rural areas.

Within China's health service system, the CDCs, maternal and child health facilities, community health-care services, and over half of all hospitals are public institutions. These public institutions are usually set up according to administrative areas, for example, CDC system includes its agencies at national, provincial, prefecture (city), and district (county) levels, while that of maternal and child health facilities include its agencies at provincial, city, district, and county levels. In terms of institutional function, there is little overlap between CDCs and hospitals; however, maternal and child health facilities have overlapping functions with both CDCs and hospitals [7].

3.3   Public Health Education

Over a 100 years, China's public health education has experienced several phases. Great numbers of public health professionals were trained and joined China's public health work. During these phases, the name of the discipline changed from "preventive medicine" to "public health and preventive medicine," with more colleges qualified to provide academic programs and capable of recruiting more students; and the curriculum has changed from purely biomedicine to the combination of biomedicine with social science, with graduates working in increasingly multiple careers. Entering twenty-first century, China has established a well-structured and multilevel public health professional training system which is able to deliver a huge number of public health workforce. Nowadays, China's public health education has shouldered the mission of cultivating highly qualified professionals with the objective of protecting and promoting health for the entire Chinese population.

3.3.1   The Beginning (1907–1949)

In 1907, Dr. Junges, a German, began to teach a course on hygiene at the Shanghai German Medical School. The School of Hygiene then was set up in 1913. In 1914, the private West China Union University launched a "hygiene and health science" course for its medical students. The university also established a department of hygiene in 1936. In 1921, John B. Grant at the Peking Union Medical College (PUMC) embarked on his public health work. In 1932, Chen Zhiqian and his colleagues piloted the famous "Ding County Model" that focused on health education as well as public health practices [8]. This pilot at the grassroots level was implemented more than four decades earlier than WHO-proposed "Health for all in 2000" (1977). The Ding County Model was promoted widely around the world, especially in developing nations. After the Anti-Japanese War broke out in 1931, large numbers of refugees and casualties led to a high incidence of infectious diseases. Medical schools within comprehensive universities in major cities like Peking (Beijing today), Shanghai, and Chongqing subsequently established department of hygiene and recruited a small number of students. In 1940, the China Medical University in Yan'an launched a preventive medicine program and trained a group of public health professionals, which laid the foundation for the development of preventive medicine education afterward.

3.3.2   Development and Discontinuation (1950–1978)

In the early days of the People's Republic of China, Chinese people were mired in poverty and diseases after having gone through the ravages of war. There were widespread outbreaks of various diseases, and large numbers of professionals were needed to undertake prevention and control efforts. In August 1950, at the inaugural National Health Conference jointly organized by the Ministry of Health and the Department of Health of Central Military Commission, the guiding principles for China's health policy were confirmed as follows: "serving the workers, farmers and soldiers; prevention first; integration of traditional Chinese medicine and Western medicine." Since then, the "prevention first" approach became a basic principle to guide China's health policy. Subsequently, departments of hygiene were established in ten colleges, including China Medical University, Beijing Medical College, Shanghai Medical College, and Sichuan Medical College. Take Beijing Medical College as an example, the department of hygiene included six teaching groups: epidemiology, maternal and child health, applied nutrition, biostatistics, health education, and school hygiene. In 1952, the department was reorganized based on the former Soviet Union's experience in the teaching of preventive medicine, with the establishment of six divisions: epidemiology, environmental and occupational health science, maternal and child health, applied nutrition, health administration and health education, and medical statistics. In August 1954, the Ministry of Health held the 10th National Meeting on Higher Medical Education, confirming a 5-year program of preventive medicine starting from 1955. In early 1955, the Ministry of Health decided to consolidate the nine universities which had the departments of hygiene into six universities. In the same year, six departments were established according to the six major administrative regions of the country: department of hygiene in Beijing Medical College, department of hygiene in Harbin Medical College, department of hygiene in Shanxi Medical College, department of hygiene in Shanghai First Medical College, department of hygiene in Wuhan Medical College, and department of hygiene in Sichuan Medical College. A total of 1702 students were admitted to study the science of hygiene across the country that year. In 1958, during "the Great Leap Forward," departments of hygiene were established in medical colleges in all 17 provinces and municipalities across the country. By the summer of 1962, these 17 departments were closed, with only the original 6 remaining until 1966. The "Cultural Revolution" between 1966 and 1976 saw severe destruction on the education of hygiene and others; undergraduate programs were changed to 3 years, while the number of enrollment decreased. In addition, the syllabus and teaching materials were also reduced and deleted. As there was a severe lack of health professionals, after 1973 a small number of medical colleges in certain provinces and municipalities began to launch hygiene programs and recruit students [9].

3.3.3 Recovery and Reconstruction (1978–2000)

The university entrance examination system was restored across China in 1978, and a new era began for the education of hygienic studies. Following the beginning of reform and opening up, the field began to develop rapidly, with teaching standards in the original six departments of hygiene improved continuously. In 1981, the Sichuan Medical College launched a health inspection program nationwide, while the Wuhan Medical College launched an environmental health program.

The medical colleges were upgraded to universities since 1985, with departments upgraded to schools of public health at the same time. In April 1985, the department of hygiene in Harbin Medical University was upgraded to the School of Public Health, which included 4 majors (hygiene, health inspection, health management, and nutrition and nutritional health) with a total of 15 divisions. Subsequently, Beijing Medical University, Shanghai Medical University, West China Medical University, and Tongji Medical University all had their departments of hygiene upgraded into schools of public health. All the other medical colleges around the country also began to establish departments or schools of public health of their own. By 1995, the number of schools/departments of public health increased to 41 around the country with a total of 5753 students enrolled. Master programs were also available at these faculties and schools. In 1993, the first cohort of doctoral students of public health and preventive medicine was enrolled. By 1998, a total of 648 master students and 32 doctoral students had graduated from public health and preventive medicine degree programs in China. In the early 1990s to 2000, China's institutions of higher medical education have undergone a series of changes, from scale to organizational setup. In particular, in 2000, many independent medical universities merged with comprehensive universities. The Beijing Medical University merged into Peking University, while the Shanghai Medical University merged into Fudan University. The West China Medical University merged into Sichuan University. Tongji Medical University, the Central China Science and Technology University, and the Wuhan City Construction Institute merged to form the Huazhong University of Science and Technology. The schools of public health at these institutions have subsequently become integral parts of these comprehensive universities.

3.3.4   Opportunities and Development (2000–)

In 2000, after 20 years' economic reform, China urgently need large numbers of high-quality professionals in public health management, especially after the 2003 SARS crisis, with the topic of "public health" becoming well known to every house-hold. The number of enrolled students also increased correspondingly (Table 3.1). In 2000, a total of 2675 students were admitted to postgraduate programs in

Table 3.1 Enrollment of students in preventive medicine and clinical medicine (2000–2010)

Year	Clinical medicine	Preventive medicine
2000	89,468	2675
2002	105,815	3164
2005	147,726	4417
2006	155,242	4641
2008	175,221	5239
2009	202,892	6066
2010	219,549	6565

preventive medicine, while this figure expanded by 2.5 times to 6565 in 2010. The rise was particularly dramatic between 2002 and 2005, when the figure grew from 3164 to 6066. In addition, over 1000 students annually were enrolled in health inspection programs. As the demand for health inspection professionals was huge, some universities have expanded the enrollment [5].

By the end of 2013, preventive medicine programs were offered in 84 colleges and universities across China. The undergraduate program was generally 5 years in accordance with Ministry of Education stipulations. Students who completed the programs successfully were awarded Bachelor of Medicine. In certain schools, students were given a 5–7-year flexible timeframe to complete their studies. In these programs, students mainly undertook courses in basic medicine, clinical medicine, and preventive medicine and trained with the basic methodology in terms of medical research design, statistical analysis, biomedical testing, and disease prevention and control techniques, to build their capacity on the prevention and control of infectious disease and occupational disease, environmental health, food safety surveillance and monitoring, and health management. In addition, over 60 colleges and universities offer programs in health inspection or preventive medicine programs with specializations in health inspection. In 2012, the Ministry of Education once again made adjustments to undergraduate subject catalogue, recategorizing the major of health inspection under the medical technologies category. The name of the discipline was also changed to health inspection and quarantine. Students who successfully completed the 4-year program were awarded Bachelor of Science. Universities can practice a 4–5-year flexible timeframe according its own situation. Due to many adjustments in the discipline of health inspection by the Ministry of Education over the years, universities have different polices in terms of disciplinary classification, systems, and degrees awarded.

3.3.5 Current Situation and Challenges

China's public health education has, over the 100 years, developed into a multilevel structure comprised of undergraduate, master, and PhD students. By the end of 2016, 93 colleges and universities offer 5-year bachelor's degree programs in preventive medicine. The 5-year undergraduate program characterized by a four-phase design is the main body of China's public health education. The four phases contain general education, basic medical courses, clinical medicine, and public health education. Bachelor degree of medicine is awarded after graduation. Basic medicine, clinical medicine, and preventive medicine are the major disciplines offered in most universities, including the core courses such as epidemiology, health statistics, health education, occupational health, environmental health, nutrition and food safety science, health management, toxicology, child and adolescent health, and maternal health. A total of 13 universities are authorized to offer doctoral degree programs in public health. Over 40 public health schools have launched part-time and full-time Masters in Public Health (MPH) programs, and these schools recruit 7000 students for undergraduate courses, 1500 students for master courses, and 400 students for doctoral courses each year. Graduates mostly work in CDCs, health inspection and law enforcement agencies, medical institutions, environment protection agencies, entry-exit inspection and quarantine agencies, research institutes, colleges and universities, health administrative departments, and private sectors [10].

With rapid development of science and technology, profound changes have taken place in mankind production and lifestyle, as well as in human environment. Industrialization, urbanization, information technology, globalization, and population aging—all these changes have imposed unprecedented challenges on public health. Health impacts are also the results of climate change, ecological change, environmental deterioration, food safety issues, occupational hazards, and terrorism and also concerning the double burden of emerging infectious diseases and chronic noncommunicable diseases. In such a complex situation, we have to think deeply how to cultivate high-quality public health professionals who can adapt to rapid social reform, so that they will be able to deal with these global health challenges more effectively.

3.4   Science and Technology of Public Health

3.4.1   Studies on Prevention and Control of Infectious Diseases

Among 6 billion people in the world, approximately 1500 die every hour due to infectious diseases. The majority of these 1500 deaths occur in developing countries. With China's social economic development, ecological changes, and the changing mechanism of social employment and distribution, new patterns of infectious diseases have emerged. Diseases that were previously under control, such as tuberculosis and polio, have also re-emerged; key infectious diseases such as AIDS, hepatitis, and hemorrhagic fever continue to be active with rising incidence rates, and these diseases have potential risks of epidemic outbreaks. New infectious diseases—like SARS and avian influenza—continue to emerge. To address the situation of these infectious diseases, research studies covering various topics have been conducted, such as epidemiological characteristics and gene mutation patterns of key infectious diseases; evaluation on the effectiveness of large-scale immunization with vaccines for key infectious diseases; identifying and diagnostic techniques and diagnostic reagents, especially rapid diagnostic techniques for key infectious diseases; development of new vaccines for infectious diseases; etc.

3.4.2   Studies on Prevention and Control of NCDs

In China, 80% of all deaths and 86% of the disease burden can be attributed to NCDs. Each year, around six million people die of tobacco exposure, while another 3.2 million die from lack of exercise. At the same time, approximately 2.3 million people die of harmful use of alcohol. Unhealthy diets have led to a rise in the incidence of cardiovascular diseases and tumors, and each year, at least 2.8 million persons die of obesity-related diseases. Hypercholesterolemia is the major cause of another 2.6 million deaths. Cancer-related infections also cause at least another two million deaths annually. Furthermore, these risk factors continue to be on the rise; the upward trend in morbidity of NCDs has not been curbed effectively. To address these NCD challenges, studies covering the following topics have been conducted: studies on the epidemiology and distribution of chronic diseases; studies on the etiology of chronic diseases and risk factors; large-scale population studies and the establishment of biological specimen bank to explore the etiology of chronic diseases; cohort studies focused on special population (such as birth cohort, twin cohort) and specific chronic disease patients; community-based comprehensive prevention and control demonstration projects; and studies on the monitoring of chronic diseases and the assessment of the health economics of chronic diseases, etc.

3.4.3 Studies on Environment and Health

The ecological model in public health indicated that human health is closely related to the living environment. In recent years, these tragedies happened frequently— natural disasters, extreme weather events, and environmental pollution incidents, emerging and re-emerging of certain infectious diseases, and all kinds of hazards— all related to the environment that we live in. To address these issues, studies covering the topics have been conducted: hygiene studies on air, water, and soil; special research on air pollution, such as studies on PM2.5 particulates; studies on heavy metal contamination of the soil; studies on safe drinking water and water pollution; studies on the ecological environment and changes in the environment; and studies on the building and assessment of the built environment, etc.

3.4.4 Studies on Evidence-Based Public Health Policy

The application of evidence-based medicine in health care has gained great importance, which gradually expand to other areas. Public health services should be efficient and equitable; also the public has increasing demand for an open and transparent government. It requires that the development of the public health policies should shift from the conventional model on the basis of political factors, social opinions, and economic conditions, as well as the free will of the policy-makers, to a new model based on scientific evidence. Therefore, progress has been made rapidly in recent years in the studies of evidence-based health policy-making, public health information technology and its application, generation and application of evidence on health and health economics [11].

Six decades has seen rapid growth of China's medical science and technology, with more and more plans and projects at national level launched, for example, the

National Population and Health Project, the National Science and Technology Major Project (research on infectious diseases and the development of drugs with China's own intellectual property rights), the national-level 973 and 863 programs, the National Science and Technology Support Projects, major programs under the National Natural Science Foundation of China, and major programs in health sector, etc. National-level plans and projects have vigorously promoted the intensive studies of the research in medical science, produced fruitful results, and facilitated wide application of appropriate technologies; significant improvements have been made on the quantity and quality of academic papers which produced far-reaching influence in China and abroad. In the 10 years between 2002 and 2012, China's scientists published a total of 1.0226 million articles in international publications, ranking the second in the world in terms of the number of articles published. Articles by Chinese researchers have been cited on a total of 6.6534 million times, ranking sixth in the world and one place higher compared to the previous year; on average, each article was cited 6.51 times, a 4.8% increase over the previous year. Although this figure was still significantly lower than the global average of 10.60, the growth rate was fast. In the span of 10 years, among the manuscripts published in international publications authored by Chinese scientists, there are 14 disciplines that the number of times being cited was among the top 10 in the world [12].

3.5   Public Health Practice: Chinese Experience

Chinese experience in public health can be highlighted in a few key points: political commitment and policy support; population-based strategy and prevention first; social mobilization and community participation; appropriate technology and science and technology support; mass prevention and control; and funding support. To explain these points further:

(1) Public health is a social welfare. It is indispensable of government leadership and support, as well as a favorable policy and legislation environment.
(2) The principle of "prevention first" has been highlighted in the 60 years' development of China's public health, and the preventive population-based approach has been proved to be an effective measure to reduce the incidence of diseases.
(3) Public health is an undertaking for the health of all, which involves various sectors such as health, agriculture, environmental protection, education, and technology; it needs social mobilization and multi-sectoral coordination and also needs community participation to raise public awareness and take actions to promote health.
(4) With the socioeconomic development, and the advancement of science and technology, public health is also exploring new knowledge and technology, hoping to apply these evidence-based, appropriate technologies to improve population health.

(5) The concerns by the government and all circles of society and the financial investment are the basic safeguards for a sustainable development of public health.

3.5.1 Prevention First

The principle of "prevention first" has been a mainstay of China's public health work. It is a highly summarized and scientific conclusion of China's public health experience. Its implementation has been well-recognized by Chinese people, and this cost-effective strategy has become an important integral part of China's health development with its characteristics. The building of public health institutions and teams, the transformation of basic sanitation facilities in both urban and rural areas, and the implementation of large-scale immunization programs have all helped China to efficiently keep infectious disease under control. Smallpox was eradicated in 1963, while the target of "polio-free" was realized in 2000. In numerous disaster relief and disease prevention operations, the commitment to the "prevention first" approach and the implementation of disease surveillance, epidemic reporting, incident handling, food hygiene supervision, environmental monitoring, etc., in accordance with disease prevention plans, have helped to prevent outbreaks in the wake of major disasters. All these have played positive role in ensuring physical and mental health of Chinese people and promoting the steady development of the society.

3.5.2 Government Leadership, Multi-sectoral Coordination, and Community Participation

The strategy that governments at various levels are responsible for all aspects of public health work, for mobilizing all forces from community groups and organizations, and for mobilizing community participation, is a key strategy contributing to the booming development of public health since the founding of new China in 1949, which is also the basis of the implementation of the "prevention first" principle. The work of disease prevention and control falls under public welfare in China, that is, such work is performed in service of the whole society and all people; this in turn means that the development of public health in China must be spearheaded by the government and requires coordination between various sectors as well as the broad participation of the whole of society. Practice has shown that the key contributing factors for the significant achievements made in public health to date align with the distinctive characteristics of Chinese public health efforts. Since the reform and opening-up policy was introduced, the Chinese government has regarded the work of disease prevention and control as a key part of building up socialist culture in China. As such, the government established the basic policy of "organization by the government; responsibility by local governments; coordination between agencies; mobilization of the masses;

science-based management; and monitoring by society," leading public health efforts along the way to be more regularized, institutionalized, standardized, and legalized.

3.5.3   Public Health Legislation

Since the founding of new China in 1949, especially after the reform and opening up in late 1970s, China has stepped up the pace in terms of establishing the legal foundation for public health and has basically formed the corresponding legal system and supervision system. Currently, 10 health legislations have been passed by the Standing Committee of the National People's Congress, and 27 sets of regulations have been issued by the State Council. These laws and regulations include the Law of the People's Republic of China on the Prevention and Treatment of Infectious Diseases, the Frontier Health and Quarantine Law, the Food Safety Law, the Law of the People's Republic of China on Maternal and Infant Health Care, the Law of the People's Republic of China on Blood Donation, the Law on Licensed Doctors, the Law of the People's Republic of China on Prevention and Control of Occupational Diseases, Regulations on the Administration of Public Health Venues, Regulations on the Prevention and Control of Pneumoconiosis, Regulations on the Supervision and Management of AIDS, Regulations on Radiation Protection Against Radioactive Isotopes and Radiation Devices, Regulations on the Health Monitoring of Cosmetic Products, Regulations on Campus Health Work, Management Regulations for the Addition of Iodine to Table Salt to Eradicate Iodine Deficiency, Regulations for the Management of Blood Products, etc. [13].

The Ministry of Health has further issued over 400 detailed rules based on the above. Local people's congresses and governments have also issued a large volume of local-specific rules and regulations in line with local conditions. China has preliminarily established a hygiene and health standards system that is compatible with local conditions and also in line with the best global standards. Statistics show that there are over 1300 sets of hygiene and health standards in place in China, covering potable water, food safety, cosmetic product safety, the safety of sterilized products, hygienic standards in public venues, occupational health, school health, protection against radiation, food and cosmetics testing methods, and the diagnosis of food poisoning and cosmetics-induced skin ailments, etc. In addition, we have also established a series of standard hygienic practices, as well as safety and functional assessment methods and procedures that have essentially met the needs for disease prevention and control and public health inspection in China.

3.5.4   Decentralization and Delegation

Given China's large population, vast land area, complex landscape, and disparities in socioeconomic development between regions, the central government cannot take full charge of public health as well as other efforts.

The well-organized and coordinated development of public health work will only be possible with a reasonable division of responsibilities between the central and local governments, as this would give full play to the capabilities of both. One long-standing principle is that the central government, which spearheads public health efforts nationwide, is responsible for developing health legislation and regulations, policies, and national plans. The central government is also responsible for providing guidance and coordinating solutions for key health issues on the national or trans-regional level, as well as for adopting multiple methods to help local governments improve their public health practice. On the other hand, local governments take full responsibilities for public health programs conducted within their respective areas, integrate public health agenda into the overall social and economic development plans of that area, and establish standards for the allocation of health resources according to health planning guidelines from the central government. The local government is also responsible for the implementation of health plans at the local level. The central government provides local governments with targeted guidance based on specific circumstances such as region and characteristics and depending on the area of expertise involved. This approach has seen significant improvements in the health levels of the people in various areas and across different social groups, meaning that the "health for all" strategy has been truly implemented and has yielded positive results.

3.5.5   Patriotic Health Campaign

Patriotic health campaign, an innovation of China's socialist health development, is a working approach characterized by government leadership and multi-sectoral cooperation, mobilizing all society to join public health efforts. Over the last few decades, patriotic health campaign has made far-reaching impacts in terms of promoting social change, improving urban and rural cleanliness, and enhancing health knowledge and health levels of the people.

Prior to the reform and opening up, its focus was on cleaning up of rural and urban environments on a regular basis. Following economic reform and social economic development, its priorities expanded. In the rural areas, local governments at various levels have integrated the improvement of water and sanitation into the local development plan, and made necessary arrangement for the implementation, which became the basis and foundation of the "moderately prosperous society" that 900 million rural residents look forward to. By the end of 2004, a total of 886.156 million people (including 7.724 million people in the current year) nationwide have benefited from tap water programs, accounting for 93.8% of the total rural population, and 60.0% of the rural population have access to tap water. A total of 131.924 million rural households utilized improved sanitation, including 3.394 million households who installed improved sanitation in 2004; in total, 53.1% of the rural population have access to the improved sanitation. The sewage treatment rate is 57.5%. Significant achievements have been made with the water and sanitation improvement programs, which have effectively protected the health of rural residents [14]. In the urban areas, "hygienic cities," "hygienic towns," and "hygienic workplaces" have been built, in order to upgrade the urban infrastructure, to manage the air pollution, and to improve social culture for creating a healthy living and working environment for the urban population; and assessments are organized to evaluate the outcome.

These practices have greatly contributed to the city's overall health development and produced a profound impact on the improvement of cities' investment environment, economic development, people's health awareness, and civilization progress.

3.5.6   Public Health Infrastructure and Human Resources

Originally, public health institutions in China were organized along the lines of the country's administrative districts. These institutions include epidemic prevention stations and maternal and child care centers at the provincial, city, and county levels which were led by health administrations at the same level and which received technical guidance from institutions one level above. Public health institutions below the county level include preventive health-care departments in hospitals of various levels, epidemic prevention teams in township hospital and independent preventive health-care clinics, health clinics within mining enterprises and manufacturing plants, and campus clinics. By the end of 2004, there were a total of 3586 CDCs (including 135 preventive health-care centers) around the country, and 1279 health inspection institutes at various levels, and there were also 14,000 community health centers (stations) and 2997 maternal and child health centers (stations). The CDCs (and epidemic prevention stations) employed a total of 210,000 public health professionals, including 36,505 professionals in health inspection institutes [15].

China's public health team is comprised of many devoted and dedicated professionals with strong technical expertise, fulfilling the tasks of disease prevention and control, health surveillance and monitoring, health education, maternal and child health care, and applied research and training. They play a critical role in the prevention and control of infectious diseases and endemic diseases, in maternal and child health care, in handling of health emergencies, and in the wake of numerous disasters where disease prevention was a priority. As such, they have made important contribution to social stability, economic development, and population health.

In particular, the three-tiered rural health service delivery system comprised of county, township, and village health facilities, as an important component of China's health service delivery system, has ensured the accessibility of basic health-care services for the vast rural population and has played multiple functions and provided comprehensive services. With the three-tiered health service network, the rural population can seek medical treatment for minor diseases in the village and for major diseases in the county. The practices of disease prevention and control as well as the clinical treatment at grassroots health facilities have become an important vehicle for China's implementation of primary health-care system, which can ensure the availability and accessibility of the rural population to health-care services.

China's health inspection professionals, working in the areas of prevention and control of infectious diseases, food safety, occupational safety, radiation health, environmental health, and school health, have also made outstanding contribution to the improvement of population health and promotion of public health development.

3.5.7   Preventive Strategy of Immunization

Immunization is a low-cost and highly effective means of preventing infectious diseases, and it is a fundamental task in the area of public health. The Chinese government attaches great importance to the child health and thus also attaches great importance to the immunization program.

For 50 years, China's immunization strategy has experienced a shift from "emergency immunization" to "planned immunization." Vaccinia (smallpox) inoculation was conducted free of charge across China in the early 1950s. At the same time, immunization with the BCG and DPT vaccines—against tuberculosis and diphtheria, pertussis and tetanus, respectively—were also launched. After the 1960s, China successfully developed the OPV and MV vaccines for polio and measles, respectively. The post-1949 immunization program had begun with efforts to prevent smallpox, and domestically produced vaccines were used to successfully eliminate the scourge of smallpox 16 years before the disease was declared as eradicated around the world. China has also developed vaccines against measles, poliomyelitis, diphtheria, whooping cough, tetanus, tuberculosis, Japanese encephalitis, meningococcus infection, hepatitis A, hepatitis B, rubella, chickenpox, etc., thus meeting the needs of prevention efforts against key infectious diseases of children in China. The development, promotion, and application of these vaccines have significantly reduced morbidity and mortality and led to the effective control of infectious diseases. The control of infectious diseases in China, especially the dramatic reduction in the number of cases of infectious respiratory diseases, can be attributed to the strategy of mass immunization to a large extent. The Chinese government worked with UNICEF in the early 1980s to launch cold-chain pilots in five provinces with warmer weather (Guangxi, Yunnan, Sichuan, Hubei, and Fujian) with a total population of eight million people. In 1985, the cold-chain project was expanded to cover 14 provinces and autonomous regions with a total population of 180 million. In 1986, the project was once again expanded to cover 30 provinces, autonomous regions, and municipalities with a total population of 1.03 billion, with basic cold-chain equipment prepared for over 2600 counties, local cities, and regions. Over the course of this process, the fundamental change was a shift from emergency immunization in the winter and spring to the establishment of regular immunization schedules (including weekly, every 3 months, monthly, every 2 months) for both urban and rural areas. The goal of an 85% immunization rate was first achieved at the provincial level in 1988 and then at the county level in 1990 and then at the township level in 1990. The eradication of polio was subsequently confirmed in

2000. In 2002, routine immunization rates continued to stay at a very high level. The BCG immunization rate reached 98.0%, while the immunization rate of OPV3 vaccine reached 98.2%. Immunization rate for the MV vaccine and the DPT3 vaccine was 98.4% and 97.9%, respectively.

References

1. Li L, Jiang Q. Theory and practice of public health in China. Beijing: People's Medical Publishing House; 2015.
2. Zhu A, Wu Y, Ye Y. Revitalize the cooperative medical care system. Chin Rural Health Serv Adm. 1991;11(12):19–24.
3. Liu J, Han W. To revitalize rural health work, we must adhere to four principles. Chin Health Serv Manag. 1998;15(3):135–7.
4. Zhang L, Hu Z, Chen S. Health care management. Beijing: People's Medical Publishing House; 2013.
5. National Bureau of Statistics. China statistical summary 2014. Beijing: China Statistics Press; 2014.
6. Du Y. Maternal and child health management. Beijing: Peking Union Medical College Press; 2012.
7. Wang Y, Yang G. Public health in China. Beijing: Peking Union Medical College Press; 2013.
8. Chen Z. The main thoughts of Professor Chen Zhiqian in the Model of Ding County. Mod Prev Med. 2004;31(5):651–3.
9. Li L. Challenges facing public health in China in the 21st century, and countermeasures. Chin J Health Educ. 2003;19(1):5–7.
10. Nan C, Jun L, Liming L. Comparative study on master of public health (MPH) education between China and America. Mod Prev Med. 2008;35(15):2893–5.
11. Brownson RC, Baker EA, Leet TL, et al. Evidence-based public health. Oxford: Oxford University Press; 2011.
12. China Science and Technology Paper Statistics and Analysis Research Group. 2012 China science and technology paper statistics and analysis bulletin. Chin J Sci Tech Periodicals. 2014;25(1):27–34.
13. Wang J. Health law. 4th ed. Beijing: People's Medical Publishing House; 2013.
14. National Bureau of Statistics. China rural statistical yearbook 2005. Beijing: China Statistics Press; 2005.
15. Ministry of Health. China health statistics yearbook 2005. Beijing: Peking Union Medical College Press; 2005.

Public Health Challenges in China

Liming Li, Xiaosong Li, and Bo Wang

In the twenty-first century, with the rapid social economic development, the process of industrialization, urbanization, and population aging has led to the changes of disease pattern, ecologic environment, and lifestyle. China is now facing a complex situation with health threats from multiple diseases and various health determinants, which are the similar difficult issues that both the developed and developing countries have to deal with. Specifically, the challenges in China cover the following perspectives: demographic changes, double burden of diseases due to changes of disease spectrum, the negative effects of industrialization and urbanization, food and drug safety issues, public health emergencies, and health inequities [1].

4.1 Demographic Changes

4.1.1 Population Aging

An aging population is a pressing challenge in China, which has the characteristics of large-scale, rapid pace, and uneven distribution between regions. By the end of 2014, the population above 60 years of age has reached 212 million, accounting for 15.5% of the total population. It is estimated that the number will reach 308 million, 21.1% of the total population in 2025 [2]. The aging issue has posed an increasing

L. Li (✉)
School of Public Health, Peking University, Beijing, China
e-mail: lmlee@vip.163.com

X. Li
West China School of Public Health, Sichuan University, Chengdu, Sichuan, China

B. Wang
Meinian Institute of Health, Beijing, China

© Springer Nature Singapore Pte Ltd. and People's Medical Publishing House, PR of China 2019
L. Li, Q. Jiang (eds.), *Introduction to Public Health in China*, Public Health in China,
https://doi.org/10.1007/978-981-13-6545-4_4

demand for the aged healthcare, which also brings severe challenges to China's healthcare services and social security system. The 4th National Health Service Survey shows that 50% of the aged in China are NCD patients, and that number increases to 64.5% among the aged above 65; the proportion of NCD patients rises with aging process, so is the proportion of aged whose daily life is affected by NCDs [3]. What's more challenging is that China is now in an aging society that is "getting old before getting rich." An increase in absolute and relative numbers of aging population imposes heavy burden on the society as a whole, resulting in huge pressure on the resources of social security.

4.1.2 Demographic Dividend Disappearing

The term "population dividend" refers to a high proportion of working people in the total population with a low dependency ratio, indicating a positive structure of population age which contributes to the economic growth. After over three decades' implementation of the one-child policy, China is now seeing a trend with aging population, low birth rates, decreased population growth, and a declining proportion of workforce. The population dividend is disappearing as a result. The aging of the population and the rapid decline in the proportion of young workforce have had a serious impact on labor supply and the relevant social savings and capital accumulation, thus limiting future economic growth. This reality requires us to place greater emphasis on protecting and improving the health of the working population as well as enhancing labor productivity.

4.2 Double Burden of Disease

4.2.1 Emerging and Reemerging Infectious Diseases

New infectious diseases such as the H1N1 influenza, a highly pathogenic avian influenza in humans, the West Nile fever, the Middle East respiratory syndrome (MERS), and Ebola are typically zoonotic diseases that are transmitted in a variety of ways at great speeds. These diseases also typically mutate more quickly and are capable of infecting large numbers of people easily. Under the background of globalization, modern air, land, and sea transportation networks make it even easier for infectious diseases to spread around the world. This poses serious threats to the health of the Chinese people [4]. For instance, the H1N1 influenza pandemic that originated in Mexico in March 2009 spread to over 200 countries in the world in the short span of the few months, causing tens of thousands of deaths. Global tourist numbers fell by 25–30%, with economic losses of over USD2 trillion reported [5].

Reemerging infectious diseases are diseases that had been previously controlled but have seen a resurgence in recent years in certain countries and regions, including tuberculosis, malaria, cholera, dengue fever, yellow fever, and diphtheria. The reemergence of these diseases and variation of pathogens can be attributed to factors such as drug resistance, the weakening of public health efforts, urbanization and globalization, the lack of health and other basic infrastructure, and climate change. This is another serious threat to the health of Chinese people. To take tuberculosis as an example, China is one of 22 TB high-burden countries in the world. A million new cases are reported yearly, with approximately 100,000 cases being multidrug-resistant TB (MDR-TB) and 10,000 of extensively drug-resistant TB (TDR-TB) cases [6].

4.2.2   Chronic Noncommunicable Diseases (NCDs) and Injuries

In 2012, 86.6% of all deaths reported in China were caused by NCDs. Both mobility and mortality due to NCDs continue to rise every year, with the disease burden accounting for 68.7% of the country's total disease burden [7]. Noncommunicable diseases are chronic diseases of long duration, slow progression, and wide prevalence, costly and high rates of disability and mortality, imposing heavy burden on China's socioeconomic development. The current burden of NCDs is a reflection of the exposure level of risk factors in the past, and the future burden of NCDs is determined by the current exposure level. Currently in China, the risk factors for NCDs continue to rise: there are more than 300 million smokers in China, and 52.9% of Chinese men aged 15 years and older smoke, while 72.4% of non-smokers are exposed to secondhand smoking; in 2012, on average, every person aged 18 or older drinks 3 L of pure alcohol per year, with 9.3% of drinkers being exposed to harmful use of alcohol; in 2012, the average daily salt intake of every person was 10.5 g, much more than WHO recommended 5 g; in 2013, only 18.7% of Chinese adults aged 20–69 did regular exercises; in 2012, 30.1% of all adults aged 18 and older were overweight, and 11.9% were obese; and the prevalence of high blood pressure among Chinese aged 18 and older in 2012 was 25.2% and that of abnormal blood lipids was 32.3% [7].

Injury, which causes varying degrees of trauma, disability, and premature death, consumes huge medical resources and weakens national productivity, especially in impoverished rural areas; it makes poverty alleviation efforts even more challenging. Injury has already become one of the constraints to China's sustained economic development. In 2014, the mortality rate from injuries stood at 49.70 per 100,000 in China, with around 650,000 persons dying from injury [1]. Injury-related death has ranked fifth among all death causes, accounting for 7.67% of total deaths, and stands as the leading cause of death among people aged 1–44. The mortality rate from injury for males is 2.14 times than that for females; mortality rate of males is also higher than that of females across all age groups. The top five causes of death due to injury are similar in both urban and rural areas, which are, in order: traffic accidents, falls, suicide, drowning, and poisoning [8].

4.3 Negative Effects of Industrialization and Urbanization

China's rapid growth of industrialization and urbanization has brought about considerable environmental costs, such as the pollution of air, water, and soil [4]:

1. Air pollution: The main sources of air pollution are thermal power plants, industrial enterprises, and various engine-powered vehicles. In recent years, some regions of China have suffered from severe air pollution, with smoggy conditions becoming common weather. Particulate matter (PM) in the air is a key component of smog. PM10 particles (of diameter ≤ 10 microns) and fine PM2.5 particles (of diameter ≤ 2.5 microns) can cause health damage to the respiratory system, the cardiovascular system, the immune system, the nervous system, and the reproductive system. The WHO has already classified outdoor air pollution as a new carcinogen [9].
2. Soil contamination: Heavy metal is an outstanding contamination in the soil. It refers to some significant heavy metals of biological toxicity, including mercury, thallium, cadmium, lead, and metallic arsenic. When soil is contaminated with heavy metals, levels of heavy metals found in crops may increase. Long-term consumption of such contaminated crops can damage one's health. Persistent pesticide residues in the soil can also have a negative impact on human health via the food chain and bioconcentration.
3. Water pollution: Contaminated drinking water, severely affecting people's health, has become a major challenge in China. Biological and chemical pollution of drinking water coexist at the same time, but mainly with biologic pollution, especially in the rural areas where it is a main cause of gastrointestinal disease. Although chemical pollution of drinking water is not very common, its damage to health is more severe.

4.4 Food and Drug Safety

Food safety remains an issue of huge concern for the Chinese public over the last few years. Media reports of the food scandals such as the use of industrial alcohol in alcoholic beverages, the incidents of lean meat powders, Sudan dyes, melamine milk, etc. all have caused significant social concern and economic loss in China. Take the melamine milk as an example: melamine is a substance that is harmful to human's reproductive and urinary systems. Long-term or repeated consumption of the substance can cause renal calculus. 294,000 victims mostly infants suffered from urinary abnormality [10]. The incident has also had a severe impact on Chinese food manufacturing industry. To a certain extent, the frequent occurrence of food safety incidents in China is a reflection of inadequacies of food safety laws, food product inspection techniques, risk assessment and risk management, etc.

Major drug safety incidents have also occurred from time to time in recent years, including the poisoning of 11 individuals in Hubei from a Chinese medicine product, the deaths of 9 individuals in Guangdong due to medicine made with unapproved substitute ingredients in 2006, adverse reactions to injections of *Houttuynia cordata* also in 2006, the discovery of "fake" TCM drugs found to have adulterated with unlisted drugs, and the use of "industrial gelatin capsules" for human medicine production in Zhejiang. All these incidents greatly challenged China's drug regulation and drug safety.

4.5   Public Health Emergencies

The category of public health emergencies encompasses outbreak of major infectious diseases, adverse reactions to mass immunizations or mass drugs, outbreak of mass unknown illnesses, food poisoning, acute occupational poisoning, biologic terrorism incidents, and events that have a grave impact on public health, such as natural disasters, major accidents, and social security incidents. The frequent occurrence of natural disasters, a complex public security landscape, a weak foundation in manufacturing safety, and the increased risk of imported infectious diseases can all lead to the occurrence of public health emergencies. Currently, public health emergencies in China mostly pertain to the outbreak of infectious disease and mass food poisoning. In 2014, a total of 961 public health emergencies (excluding animal epidemics) were reported in China, including 738 incidents related to infectious disease and 160 cases with food poisoning [1]. The majority of public health emergencies involved a considerable number or even large number of individuals.

4.6   Health Inequities

In 2000, the WHO assessed the performance of health system of its 191 member states. China was ranked 188th in terms of equity in health financing [11]. There are disparities in health outcomes between urban and rural populations. In 2013, compared to urban areas, the maternal mortality rate in rural areas was higher by 1.2 per 100,000, while the infant mortality rate was higher by 6.1‰, and the mortality rate for children under 5 was higher by 8.5‰ [12]. In 2009, the average life expectancy for urban residents was 5 years longer than that for rural residents. At the same time, there are significant disparities in health outcomes between different regions, with the residents in eastern region achieving the best health outcomes, in western region the poorest, and in central area in between. Health inequities are also particularly striking with disadvantaged groups like migrant workers and the poor due to factors like poor living conditions, inadequate immunization coverage, and unhealthy lifestyles.

Despite all these challenges, new opportunities are opening up—the rapid social economic development, the deepening of the health reform, the development of the "Healthy China 2030," and the new direction for public health sciences represented by genomics, systems epidemiology, biomedical big data, research based on large population cohorts, and precision medicine, all these bring rare strategic opportunities for the public health development in future China (more details in Chap. 6).

References

1. Li L, Jiang Q. Public health in China: theory and practice. Beijing: People's Medical Publishing House; 2015.
2. Ministry of Civil Affairs of the People's Republic of China. Statistical report on social service development. http://www.mca.gov.cn/article/sj/tjgb/201506/201506158324399.shtml.
3. National Health Commission of the People's Republic of China. The 4th National Health Service survey report. http://www.moh.gov.cn/mohwsbwstjxxzx/s8211/201009/49165.shtml.
4. Chinese Preventive Medicine Association. Report of academic developments in public health and preventive medicine (2014-2015). Beijing: Chinese Science and Technology Press; 2016.
5. World Health Organization. Emergencies preparedness, response: pandemic (H1N1) 2009. https://www.who.int/csr/disease/swineflu/en/.
6. Wang B, Li L. Progress in epidemiological research. Shanghai J Prev Med. 2016;28(1):3–6.
7. Chinese Academy of Medical Sciences. China medical science and technology development report. China Science; 2016.
8. Li L, Wang J. Epidemiology, vol. I. 3rd ed. Beijing: People's Medical Publishing House; 2015.
9. World Health Organization. Outdoor air pollution a leading environmental cause of cancer deaths. http://publications.iarc.fr/Book-And-Report-Series/Iarc-Monographs-On-The-Evaluation-Of-Carcinogenic-Risks-To-Humans/Outdoor-Air-Pollution-2015.
10. Wen JG, Liu XJ, Wang ZM, et al. Melamine-contaminated milk formula and its impact on children. Asia Pac J Clin Nutr. 2016;25(4):697–705.
11. World Health Organization. World Health Report 2000-Health systems: improving performance. https://www.who.int/whr/2000/en/.
12. Li L. Reconsideration on 60 years of public health in China. Chin J Public Health Manag. 2014;30(3):311–5.

A Few Thinking About Public Health Development in China

5

Liming Li, Yu Jiang, and Jun Lv

5.1 Adherence to Government-Led Public Health Development

Public health is a social welfare undertaking, and the government takes the lead in this area given its responsibility to guarantee and provide the people's interests. The explicit goal of China's healthcare reform is to establish universal coverage that provides safe, effective, convenient, and affordable basic health services to all urban and rural residents [1]. In our opinion, China's healthcare reform has the following characteristics: establishing a health system to ensure the social welfare and fairness; emphasis on the foundation (system building), strengthening primary healthcare (human resource development) and establishing mechanisms (health service delivery and health financing); and gradually realizing equitable access to public health services. From the above, it is clear that the government attaches great importance to its leadership role in health. This provides a strong policy environment for the future development of public health in China.

5.2 Adherence to Legal Framework in Public Health

An enabling legal framework plays the fundamental role in public health work. Although China has promulgated a great number of legislation and regulations related to health, the Basic Health Law has not been formulated; hopefully it will be

L. Li (✉) · J. Lv
School of Public Health, Peking University, Beijing, China
e-mail: lmlee@vip.163.com

Y. Jiang
School of Public Health, Peking Union Medical College, Beijing, China

© Springer Nature Singapore Pte Ltd. and People's Medical Publishing House, PR of China 2019
L. Li, Q. Jiang (eds.), *Introduction to Public Health in China*, Public Health in China,
https://doi.org/10.1007/978-981-13-6545-4_5

issued in the near future. In addition, China also needs to develop healthy public polices and plan; fully implement these policies, legislation, regulations, and rules; and step up the efforts to develop standards for the health sector, which should be in line with the international standards.

5.3   Adherence to Evidence-Based Public Policy-Making

Evidence-based policy-making is a way of making decisions on health regulations, policies, and plans with regard to a group of patients, a community, or a country based on research evidence. Broadly defined, evidence-based medicine is not simply limited to evidence-based clinical trials; it also plays an important role in the area of evidence-based health policy-making [2].

Public health policies and measures need to be developed based on scientific evidence; by weighing the evidence, choices and judgment could be made, and at the same time, considerations should be given to the total economic costs for providing preventive services to the individuals and society; however, economic cost should not be the primary concern; the other factors such as values, political pressures, culture, traditions, etc. should also be taken into full consideration. Only policy decisions made on the basis of scientific evidence can be safe and reliable.

However, there are still a number of issues China has to tackle in developing evidence-based public health services [3]. The main problem is that there is limited number of original research conducted in developing countries, which means that current (and those under development) systematic reviews are of little applicability to developing countries (including China) and the systematic reviews relevant to developing countries' priority health issues are inadequate; although many interventions have been proved to be effective, it is hard to implement in low-resource settings. This needs us to strengthen the basic public health research on Chinese populations in the future, in particular, to conduct large population cohort studies to accumulate basic data, to identify the specific public health issues of Chinese population, and then to find the best solutions to address these issues.

5.4   Adherence to Prioritizing Human Resource Policy in Public Health

The idea is to get the right workers with the right skills in the right place doing the right things. According to WHO's World Health Report 2006, the first principle of human resource allocation is "suitability" [4]. Public health professionals should also be allocated with this principle, so that these professionals working in various areas, such as health service provider, management, and researcher, could all play their full potentials and also complement each other, instead of being judged by his (her) education background and professional qualifications.

5.5   Adherence to Science and Technology Strategy to Support Public Health

Public health work is very practical, with human beings as the objective of its practices; therefore, any public health endeavor should only be implemented after rigorous and scientific evaluation. So it needs strong science and technology support. In the future, the scientific research of public health should focus on the following areas [5]: basic public health research, including extra-large population cohort studies, studies on the mutation of infectious diseases, and research on the interaction between environmental/ecological change and genetic mutations; soft science research on public health; the building and applications of public health information systems; disease surveillance and reporting systems; public health incident monitoring and reporting systems; environmental and behavioral risk factor surveillance systems; pathogen-mutation surveillance systems; health enforcement and supervision systems; emergency command systems; etc.

5.6   Adherence to Scientific Assessment of Public Health Performance

One key feature of public health is that it is the public policy and a public good, and it is a service that yields social benefits over a fairly long period of time. Therefore, just how to evaluate public health services in terms of quality and quantity is a challenge. This process is the performance assessment of public health. The assessment system can be divided into several parts [6, 7]: assessment standards, performance measurement, progress report, and the quality improvement process; of these parts, performance measurement is the most challenging and can be completed through process measurement, capability measurement, outcome measurement, etc. It is imperative that we enhance the assessment of public health performance in China, as well as conduct the corresponding research.

References

1. Chinese Academy of Medical Sciences. China medical reform development report. Peking Union Medical College Press; 2016.
2. Gray M, Tang J. Evidence-based decision making in health care. Beijing: Peking University Medical Press; 2004.
3. Tang J, Li L. Some reflections on evidence-based medicine, precision medicine, and big-data research. Chin J Epidemiol. 2018;39(1):1–7.
4. World Health Organization. World health report 2006. https://www.who.int/whr/2006/en/.
5. Li L. Reconsideration on 60 years of public health in China. Chin J Public Health Manag. 2014;30(3):311–5.
6. Li L, Jiang Q. Public health in China: theory and practice. Beijing: People's Medical Publishing House; 2015.
7. Li L. Challenges facing public health in China in the 21st century, and countermeasures. Chin J Health Educ. 2003;19(1):5–7.

Prospects for Future Development

6

Liming Li and Hui Liu

Health is the foundation of all-round human development. President Xi Jinping has pointed out that it would not be possible to build a well-off society without universal healthcare. Public health is an endeavor that concerns the livelihood of people through disease prevention and health promotion. In more than six decades since 1949, China has worked extremely hard in the area of public health. To this end, it had established a developmental path that is compatible with the specific circumstances of the country and made remarkable achievements that have drawn global attention [1]. Since the 18th CPC National Congress, China has established the world's largest healthcare network, and improvements have been made in increasing the equality of basic public health services, as well as the overall capacities of public health work and the disease prevention and control.

However, various health threats still exist in China; the Party and the government decide to accelerate the process of health development, including public health. At the Fifth Plenary Session of the 18th CPC Central Committee, a decision was made to pursue the strategy of "Promotion of a Healthy China." In 2016, China held its first National Health Conference in the twenty-first century, where the outline of "Healthy China 2030" was issued, and China also hosted the 9th Global Conference on Health Promotion [2]. A blueprint for China's future health development, together with a series of strategic measures, has been confirmed.

Chinese public health professionals are called to meet the challenges and grasp the opportunities through implementing the concept of "health in life course" and

L. Li (✉)
School of Public Health, Peking University, Beijing, China
e-mail: lmlee@vip.163.com

H. Liu
Peking Union Medical College, Beijing, China

© Springer Nature Singapore Pte Ltd. and People's Medical Publishing House, PR of China 2019
L. Li, Q. Jiang (eds.), *Introduction to Public Health in China*, Public Health in China, https://doi.org/10.1007/978-981-13-6545-4_6

progressing in terms of promoting healthy lifestyle, optimizing health services, building healthy environment, and promoting global health with determination and commitment to move forward to a bright future.

6.1 New Opportunities in China

6.1.1 Multiple and Complex Threats on Health

As introduced in Chap. 4, with the rapid social economic development, the process of industrialization, urbanization, and population aging have led to the changes of disease pattern, ecologic environment, and lifestyle. China is now facing a complex situation with health threats from multiple diseases and various health determinants, which are the similar difficult issues that both the developed and developing countries have to deal with [3].

After the founding of new China in 1949, the highly infectious diseases such as cholera, smallpox, and the plague were eradicated, and in 2000 the WHO declared China polio-free; moreover, China has gained effective control over diseases such as measles, diphtheria, whooping cough, and tetanus [1]; however, the challenges to tackle other infectious diseases such as TB and AIDS still remain huge, and the risks of re-emerging infectious diseases remain high. At the same time, chronic noncommunicable diseases impose new and serious threats to public health [4, 5]. There are 260 million NCD patients in China— huge patient base, with the number increasing rapidly. NCDs cause 85% of all deaths and comprise 69% of the total disease burden in China. The rising trend of the risk factors contributing to NCDs poses a long-term and tough task for Chinese public health professionals.

China became an aging society by international standards around 1999– 2000. It is estimated that 14% of the population will be aged above 65 by 2025, making China a severely aging society by that time [3]. While life expectancy for the Chinese people is becoming longer, the health issues presented cannot be ignored. A rapidly aging society poses tremendous challenges in terms of medical services, nursing, rehabilitation, day-to-day care, community services, etc.

The level of healthy behavior and health literacy of Chinese people is still low, and there are many diseases caused by unhealthy lifestyle. Results from a 2013 study of healthy behavior show that the health literacy level of China's urban and rural residents stands at 9.48% [6]. In other words, only around one in ten residents is considered to have basic health knowledge. A 2010 study of chronic disease also shows that 83.8% of the resident population aged above 18 did not engage in any sort of physical exercises, while in 80.9% of households, salt consumption exceeded 5 g per day; in 83.4% of households, oil consumption exceeded 25 g per day, while 52.8% of residents consumed less than 400 g of fruits and vegetables daily [4]. In addition, environmental issues, safety issues, etc. also have negative impact on people's health in varying degrees.

6.1.2   Strategic Opportunities for Public Health Development

The Party and the Chinese people are providing new opportunities for the development of public health. With the rising living standards and education level, Chinese people's demand on health is increasing. In such a new situation, the Party and the government place a high priority on the improvement of people's health and decide to accelerate the building of a Healthy China. At the National Health Conference held on August 19, 2016, the "Prevention First" principle was once again emphasized, and the "Health in All Policies" was also proposed. President Xi Jinping put forward the working principles for China's health development in the new era—with grassroots as the focus, driven by reform and innovation, prevention first, integration of traditional Chinese medicine and Western medicine, health in all policies, and co-building and sharing for health—this guiding principle is raised not only for the health sector alone; it is the country's overall principle and strategy to guide China's development in health, which has laid solid political foundation for the country's health work, including the public health work.

China's public health work has entered into the critical 15 years which is full of strategic opportunities. The outline of "Healthy China 2030" released on October 25, 2016, serves as the action guidance for the country to push forward its efforts to build a healthy China in the next 15 years [2]. "Prevention first" has been repeatedly emphasized in the overall strategy, guiding principle, and the strategic objectives, as well as the specific measures and approaches. The four areas identified in the outline—maintaining mid-to-high economic growth, upgrading of the consumption structure, science and technology innovation, and the strengthening of various systems—will provide strategic support for the development of public health in the subsequent 15 years.

The outline described three steps of strategic goals for China's health development, which includes:

(1) By 2020, China will build a basic medical care system with Chinese characteristics that covers both rural and urban residents. People's health literacy continues to improve, and the health service system becomes highly efficient. Basic healthcare services and exercise services are shared by everyone. Main health indicators will be among the top of middle- and high-income countries by 2020.

(2) By 2030, the national health system will be more mature. Developments in the health industries are more coordinated. Healthcare services and protections keep improving. The health sector has become generally fair and just, and main health indicators will reach the standards of high-income countries.

(3) By 2050, a healthy China will be built that is consistent with a modern socialist country.

The outline also indicated the specific goals by 2030, which include the following: average life expectancy grows to 79 years old; 92.2% of urban and rural residents meet the National Physical Standards; 30% of Chinese people meet the health literacy standards; a total of 530 million people participate in regular physical exercises; the premature death rate achieves a decrease by 30% compared with that of 2015; while out-of-pocket spending as share of total health expenditures falls to 25%.

6.1.3 Adherence to Social Welfare as a Solid Foundation for Public Health

China's public health development is undoubtedly in need of robust financing inputs. At the same time, as a country with a billion people, China needs to deal with the issue of health equity, which is not simply a moral imperative but a matter of the expectation and opinion of the general public. Only by maintaining the social welfare nature of public health services could the basic foundation be built and the people's access to basic healthcare services be assured.

The Party and the government attach great importance to the social welfare nature of public health services. For instance, in 2016, when the government subsidized 45 yuan per capita to cover basic public health services, 30 yuan increased from that of 15 yuan in 2009; the total investment from the central government has amounted to 106.2 billion yuan [4]. The National Health Conference indicated that China would remain committed to the social welfare nature of basic healthcare so that Chinese people could have equitable access to the systematic and continuous health services which cover the prevention, treatment, rehabilitation, and health promotion.

6.2 New Concept and Objectives of "Health Through Life Course"

President Xi Jinping has emphasized the importance of adhering to the prevention first principle and the principles of combination of disease prevention and treatment through the approaches of collaboration and coordination and mass prevention and control, striving to provide health services covering all life course for the Chinese people.

The concept of "promoting health through life course" is a concept of precision: requiring us to conduct targeted interventions to address the key health issues and the risk factors at different stages of a life course [7]. According to it, prevention and control of major diseases is still critical. It is also important to target various health determinants at different stages of life, such as individual lifestyles, production and living environment and medical services, to reduce the incidence of diseases through the implementation of the prevention first principle and promotion of healthy lifestyles.

"Promoting health through life course" is a broad and comprehensive concept, requiring us to provide equitable, accessible, systematic, and sustained health services [7]: horizontally, benefiting all populations to achieve universal coverage and, vertically, covering one's whole life course to achieve a healthy lifetime. Under this concept, all populations are covered by the needed, qualified, and affordable health services, especially the health needs of women and children, the elderly, the physically disadvantaged, and those with low income which should be addressed; and priorities should be identified to strengthen the interventions for every stage of life, from infancy to the end of life, to provide whole course health services and protections in their lives.

6.3   New Blueprint for Public Health in China

6.3.1   Raising Public Awareness in Health: Promoting Healthy Lifestyles

Individual lifestyle plays a major role in one's health, so it is an effective approach for China to address health challenges through promoting a healthy lifestyle. The National Health Conference requested to promote health in a broader sense, shifting the focus from treating diseases to the improvement of people's health.

For the promotion of healthy lifestyle, three priorities need to be strengthened: health education, healthy behavior, and physical fitness. In terms of health education, it should include both improving people's health literacy and strengthening school-based health education efforts, with integrating health education into the national education system as one important component of quality education; in terms of promoting healthy behavior, there are approaches to promote healthy diet, tobacco and alcohol control, and mental health and reduce unsafe sexual behaviors and the drug harm, which can help residents develop their own healthy behaviors and habits; and in terms of improving people' s physical fitness, efforts need to be made in improving sports facilities, conducting physical activities to cover all populations, enhancing the integration between sports and healthcare, strengthening the interventions implemented by non-health sectors, and promoting the participation of the key population group in physical activities.

Some figures can vividly describe the expected outcome through promotion of healthy lifestyle [2]: for example, by 2030, universal coverage of healthy lifestyle action at the country (city, district) level will be achieved; the average daily salt consumption per capita is to be reduced by 20%, and smoking prevalence aged 15 and above would also be lowered to 20%; and the three-tiered (county-township-village) sports facility network would be established, with no less than 2.3 square meters per capita, and these facilities would be open to the public free of charge or at a low fee. At least 25% of the students across the country would meet the "excellent" physical fitness standards.

6.3.2   Focusing on the Whole Population and Through All Life Course: Optimizing Public Health and Healthcare Services

China is set to work on improving the coverage of its public health services from the three aspects: the prevention and control of major diseases, the management of family planning services, and the equalization of basic public health services.

The prevention and control of major illnesses remain a key part of public health services. Not only do we need to reduce the spread of the major infectious diseases and deal effectively with sudden outbreaks of acute infectious diseases, we also need to strengthen the integrated prevention and control of chronic noncommunicable diseases through effective implementation of the prevention strategy. By 2030, China will establish the NCD management system covering all populations through all life-course, with overall five-year survival rate of cancer increased by 15% and caries incidence for 12-year-olds kept within 25%; the sex ratio at birth would become normal, and on the basis of improving service quality, basic public health services could be equitably accessed by both urban and rural residents [2].

Health services targeted at special populations, such as adolescents and children, women and infants, the elderly, the disabled, the migrants and those with low income, would have been effectively improved. China will move forward to establishing its various systems and mechanisms, strengthening the health work in kindergartens and schools, implementing the nutrition programs for students in impoverished areas, ensuring maternal and child health, providing continued health management services and clinical services for the aged, making efforts to help the disabled people to access the rehabilitation services, giving attention to migrant health, and implementing the health and poverty alleviation program.

6.3.3 Implementing "Health in All Policies" and Promoting a Healthy Environment

President Xi Jinping has noted that a good ecological environment is the foundation of the survival and health of a human being. China will seek to build a healthy environment by focusing on the four areas [2]:

1. China will work to tackle major environmental issues that have a negative impact on people's health. With the improvement of environment quality as the core priority, efforts will be made to prevent and control the pollution of the air, soil, and water. The most rigorous ecological and environmental protection systems will be put in place with emission targets set for industry. Efforts will also be made to establish the systems of environment and health surveillance, investigation, and risk assessment as well as to accelerate the process of land greening.
2. Continue patriotic health campaign work by promoting healthy cities and healthy villages (townships). By 2030, the rural areas will be built into beautiful home gardens, neat and clean, suitable for the aged to live; universal coverage of improved sanitation facilities will be achieved; 50% of the cities in China will be certified as hygienic cities; and a group of demonstration areas for healthy cities and healthy villages (townships) will be built as well.

3. Ensure the food and drug safety: efforts are needed to implement food safety law, to improve food safety system, to strengthen food safety supervision, and to regulate every point in the food supply chain from production to consumption, so that the general public will have no worry on the safety issue of food.

4. China will work toward improving its public safety system and reducing the health threats posed by public emergency incidents. Efforts will be made to strengthen workplace safety and occupational health, to promote road safety, to prevent and reduce injuries, to improve emergency response capacity and the cross border public health system. By 2030, the capacities of public health emergency response and the emergency medical rescue will reach the same level of the developed countries.

6.3.4   Implementing Global Health Strategy

Despite rapid development in global health, tough challenges still remain: in addition to the long-lasting diseases and health issues, as well as the issue of health inequities, there are new problems caused by aging population, cross border migration, disease pattern change, changes of ecological environment, and lifestyle [3]. Over time, China has worked hard to fulfill its international obligations and participate actively in global health governance. The humanitarian efforts China has made as a big and responsible country have also garnered positive feedback from the international community.

China will make full use of bilateral cooperation mechanisms to promote health endeavors within the "Belt and Road Initiative" region, sharing its health developmental experience, promoting partnerships in health emergency response and the prevention and control of key infectious diseases, and developing public health professional development programs, etc. The outline of the "Healthy China 2030" also states that China will continue to work on South-South cooperation with the implementation of joint Sino-African public health programs and continue to send medical professionals to developing countries to support their medical services including maternal and child health and to support the establishment of disease prevention and control system [2]. China will also make full use of the national strategic dialogue mechanism to integrate health into the diplomatic agenda of big countries. China will participate actively in global health governance and play its role in the research, negotiation, and development of the international standards, protocols and guidelines to achieve an enhanced international influence and stronger voice on health issues in the world.

"The way forward may be arduous, but we start firmly from the first step." Protecting the health of the people is a system, and it is also a tough journey that requires hard work and continuous breakthrough. China's public health sector has a long way to go, but no matter how challenging the future is, Chinese stories will continue to be written into the brilliant development history of mankind.

References

1. Li L. 60 years of public health in China: achievements and prospects. Chin J Public Health Manag. 2014;30(1):3–4.
2. The CPC Central Committee and the State Council. Outline of the healthy China 2030 plan. http://www.gov.cn/zhengce/2016-10/25/content_5124174.htm.
3. Li L. Challenges facing public health in China in the 21st century, and countermeasures. Chin J Health Educ. 2003;19(1):5–7.
4. Chinese Academy of Medical Sciences. China medical science and technology development report. China Science; 2016.
5. Li L, Wang J. Epidemiology, vol. III. 3rd ed. Beijing: People's Medical Publishing House; 2015.
6. Chinese Health Education Center. 2013 Chinese residents' health literacy monitoring report. http://www.cma.org.cn/attachment/20141219/1418966791113.pdf.
7. Li L, Jiang Q. Theory and practice of public health in China. Beijing: People's Medical Publishing House; 2015.

Further Reading

Chinese Preventive Medicine Association. Report of academic developments in public health and preventive medicine (2014–2015). Beijing: Chinese Science and Technology Press; 2016.

Dai Z. A review of China's sanitary and anti epidemic system in commemoration of the 50th anniversary of the founding of the system. Chin J Public Health Manag. 2003;19(5):377–80.

Li L. Challenges facing public health in China in the 21st century, and countermeasures. Chin J Health Educ. 2003;19(1):5–7.

Li L. 60 years of public health in China: achievements and prospects. Chin J Public Health Manag. 2014;1:3–4.

Li L, Cao W. Epidemiology, vol. II. 3rd ed. Beijing: People's Medical Publishing House; 2015.

Li L, Jiang Q. Theory and practice of public health in China. Beijing: People's Medical Publishing House; 2015.

Li L, Wang J. Epidemiology, vol. III. 3rd ed. Beijing: People's Medical Publishing House; 2015.

© Springer Nature Singapore Pte Ltd. and People's Medical Publishing House, PR of China 2019
L. Li, Q. Jiang (eds.), *Introduction to Public Health in China*, Public Health in China, https://doi.org/10.1007/978-981-13-6545-4

Printed in the United States
by Baker & Taylor Publisher Services